ADVANCED PRAISE FOR EMOTIONAL HEALING AT WARP SPEED: THE POWER OF EMDR

"This riveting book reads like a novel, using intriguing stories that unravel the mystery of how EMDR works to get beyond the brain to the heart of healing the whole Self. As an actor, artist, humanitarian, and mother, I am heartened by Dr. Grand's success in healing trauma and helping people open up to new levels of creativity and performance. His breakthrough book paints a bright picture for healing in the new millennium.

JANE SEYMOUR

"*Emotional Healing at Warp Speed* introduces us to a whole new level of miraculous healing that is going to be commonplace in the new century. Share this book with all the people you care about!"

CAROL ADRIENNE, PH.D., coauthor with James Redfield of *The Celestine Prophecy: An Experiential Guide* and *The Tenth Insight: An Experiential Guide,* and author of *Find Your Purpose, Change Your Life* and *The Purpose of Your Life*

"Having witnessed Dr. Grand's success firsthand, I can tell you that he provides amazing solutions for complex performance problems. This book is a must-read for people wishing to learn how to break down self-imposed limitations and reach their very greatest potential. I highly recommend it."

RICHARD L. WILLARD III, president, International Amateur Athletic Association & Jesse Owens International Trophy Awards

"In this book, David Grand, Ph.D., invites us on a journey where one is able to learn, feel, and witness how the healing power of EMDR works. He leads with care, sensitivity, and skillfulness into the sacred mystery of the healing process. There, like in a reflection of multiples mirrors, one can experience the fascination of confronting the infinite levels of images, never being the same but always part of the same being."

MARÌA ELENA LESMI, PH.D., EMDR facilitator, Argentina, and board member of EMDR Humanitarian Assistance Programs

"In forty years of teaching acting, I have never witnessed such profound changes in an actor's ability to reach inwardly and express outwardly, with great freedom and authority, a deeper and more complex sense of his or her character's life—and this after ten minutes' work with David. His work is the wave of the future for actor training!"

GEORGE MORRISON, president of the New Actors Workshop, professor emeritus of Theatre Arts at the State University of New York, Purchase

"Emotional Healing at Warp Speed gives the reader an easy-to-grasp overview of anxiety, trauma, and the debilitating impact they have over quality of life. Dr.Grand illustrates the profound relief that EMDR can provide and shares his own personal experiences as testimony to its versatility and power. It is a must-read for anyone seeking shelter from the storm of fear and anxiety."

JANE GREER, PH.D., psychotherapist; author of *Gridlock* and *How Could You Do This to Me?*; featured on *Oprah!*, CNN, *Montel*, others; and columnist for *Redbook* online's "Let's Talk About Sex"

"In my forty years' experience as an actor, I believe EMDR is one of the most exciting and unique methods of exploring character I've ever encountered. Using EMDR under David Grand's insightful and caring guidance I achieved, in a very short period of time, a deeper emotional and psychological understanding of a character I'd been portraying, far beyond any previous experience. This book portrays EMDR as a tool of significant value to any actor seeking a more profound reality in his work."

THOMAS RYAN, actor, former cast member of *LA Law*, guest star on over 20 television series

"After reading the chapter in this book entitled "Tales from the Rails," I had tears in my eyes, but they were tears of joy knowing that over 150 railroad engineers no longer have to fight the demons that go along with Post-Accident Stress Syndrome, and I have also made a new friend and found out that EMDR is a long-lasting treatment. I found relief from my pain and stopped blaming myself after placing myself in Dr. Grand's hands and participating in EMDR. It is a lasting experience and I have made a friend for life."

BOB FRANKE, chairman of Engineers Helping Engineers, Brotherhood of Locomotive Engineers, Division 269

Emotional Healing
at
Warp Speed

THE POWER OF EMDR

DAVID GRAND, PH.D.

Harmony Books
New York

Grateful acknowledgment is made to the following for permission to reprint previously published material:

"Doctor, My Eyes" written by Jackson Browne copyright © 1970–72 Atlantic Music Corporation/Open Window Music. © Renewed & Assigned 1998 Criterion Music Corporation/Open Window Music. All rights reserved. Used by permission of Criterion Music Corporation/Open Window Music and Wixen Music Publishing, Inc. International copyright secured.

Excerpt from "Emancipation Song" by Bob Marley copyright © 1980 Fifty-Six Hope Road, Ltd./Odnil Music Ltd./Blue Mountain Music Ltd. (PRS). All rights for North and South America controlled and administered by Rykomusic, Inc. (ASCAP). All rights for the rest of the World controlled and administered by Rykomusic, Ltd. (PRS). All rights reserved. Used by permission.

BasicBooks: Excerpt from TRAUMA AND RECOVERY by Judith Lewis Herman, M.D. Copyright © 1992 by BasicBooks, A Division of HarperCollins Publishers Inc. Reprinted by permission of Basic Books, a member of Perseus Books, L.L.C.

Published by Harmony Books, New York, New York. Member of the Crown Publishing Group.

Random House, Inc. New York, Toronto, London, Sydney, Auckland
www.randomhouse.com

HARMONY BOOKS is a registered trademark and the Harmony Books colophon is a trademark of Random House, Inc.

Printed in the United States of America

Design: Susan Maksuta

Library of Congress Cataloging-in-Publication Data
Grand, David.
    Emotional healing at warp speed : the power of EMDR / by David Grand.
      p. cm.
    1. Eye movement desensitization and reprocessing.   I. Title.
  RC489.E98 G73 2001
  616.89'14—dc21

                             2001016942

ISBN 0-609-60746-4

10 9 8 7 6 5 4 3 2

To Nina and Jonathan—
the center of my universe

ACKNOWLEDGMENTS

My deepest personal thanks go to my collaborator, Richard Marek, for helping bring my voice to the pages of this professional, personal, and creative project. His wisdom, confidence, and eloquence helped illuminate myriad experiences and information.

Of course there would be no book without EMDR and there would be no EMDR without Francine Shapiro. She has been a role model and mentor with her tireless championing of healing and humanitarianism. Francine's words, "Don't give back, give forward," have served as a beacon for me every day.

Thank you to Robbie Dunton for her invaluable reinforcement of my efforts in the "EMDR World." Robbie and Francine are the heart and soul (interchangeable) of EMDR, protecting and nurturing it for all who practice and receive it.

Appreciation to Lisa Roina, who opened the doors of ICM and has supported me each step of the way. Thanks to my literary agent, Mitch Douglas, who has ably pulled together the disparate elements of this project with skill and warmth.

Special thanks to my editor, Peter Guzzardi, whose efforts have made this book possible by seeing its viability and then helping shape it throughout the entire process. Gratitude to the staff of Crown/Harmony, especially Linda Loewenthal, Shaye Areheart, Cara Brozenich, Rhoda Dunn, and Sarah Trosper.

Thank you to my publicist, Jan Goldstoff, who insisted that I write a book and then paved the way for it. Thanks to Bob Franke for his spirit of generosity in sharing his story and teaming with me to heal countless railroad engineers. Gratitude to George Morrison for giving me my start with EMDR-based acting coaching and to Rex Knowles for his creative collaborations. Thanks to Chris Ranck and David Toney for their contributions in developing and showcasing "The Grand System." Thank you to Terrie Williams for finding new ways to apply my skills and Judith Adler for her marketing magic.

A special mention to my assistant, Laurie Delaney, for her competence and loyalty. This book would not have been possible without her tireless efforts and personal dedication. Thanks to Uri Bergmann for his friendship and for teaching me neurophysiology. Thanks to friend Carol Forgash for her encouragement and David Minshall for his wise guidance.

I want to thank my fellow EMDR facilitators, who have become my international family.

Most of all I want to thank my family. Thank-you to Nina, my soul mate, mother of our child, and my most trusted advisor; to Jonathan, my son, friend and inspiration; and to my mother and father for bringing me life and love.

CONTENTS

PART III:
ALL THE WORLD'S A STAGE:
EMDR AND PERFORMANCE ENHANCEMENT

PART IV:
THE DOORS SWING OPEN:
MY JOURNEY WITH EMDR

I
MY FIRST EXPERIENCES WITH EMDR

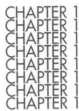

CHAPTER 1
CHAPTER 1
CHAPTER 1
CHAPTER 1
CHAPTER 1
CHAPTER 1
CHAPTER 1

CHAPTER 1   I AM INTRODUCED TO EMDR

I went without extraordinary expectations. My friend Uri Bergmann, like me a psychotherapist but more experimental than I (he was into hypnosis and pain management), had learned of a new therapeutic method called EMDR—Eye Movement Desensitization and Reprocessing. He had been impressed with the results he had achieved with it, particularly in one case, and now he wanted to learn more. He asked if I would accompany him to the Loew's Hotel on New York's Lexington Avenue for a weekend Level I training session. I somewhat reluctantly agreed.

The year was 1993. I was forty years old. My life was about to change forever.

There were about eighty of us in a conference room—several, I found out later, from abroad—all of us staring with some wonder at the striking, five-foot-eleven, dynamic, fortyish woman named Francine Shapiro who talked with confidence and clarity about the new form of psychotherapy she had developed.

I confess I didn't immediately grasp most of it. Her ideas were derived from cognitive-behavioral psychotherapy (put simplistically, what you feel comes from what you think), whereas I, trained as a psychoanalyst, believed in the influence of early life experiences in the formation of personality, conflict, and self. Her talk was highly technical, filled with words and phrases I would come to integrate only later, but I was impressed by her ardor and by the fluidity of both her words and her movements. Throughout the day, she seemed comfortable and self-assured teaching her new method.

We broke for lunch. I remember telling Uri that I was neither impressed nor unimpressed. Clearly the woman was not a wacko, and while I found it difficult to imagine myself using the approach with my own patients, I did not put down his interest. "Stick around for the experiential this afternoon," he said, though it had not occurred to me to leave.

After lunch Dr. Shapiro lectured for another hour. (Now I *was* growing restive.) We took a break, and finally the chairs in the room were rearranged, and manuals in hand, we broke into groups of three—"patient," "therapist," and "observer"—to begin what is known as the *practicum,* the hands-on session. Watching over us was a facilitator, someone already versed in EMDR practice, to guide our efforts and correct our mistakes.

Though doing the practicum with a friend is discouraged, Uri and I fortunately managed to stay together, perhaps anticipating the assignment of the third member of our group, a man in need of considerable support, who was so patently nervous that his pencil for note-taking trembled visibly in his hands. Uri and I exchanged glances, concerned with how he would perform.

Well, to begin with, he was by default the therapist, for although we were to switch roles after forty-five minutes, it fell out that for the first go-round I would be his patient and Uri the observer. Soon the facilitator arrived to give us our initial instructions. A sixtyish gentleman from Southern California with a laid-back teaching approach. I was feeling shaky. *Just my luck,* I thought. *A vulnerable therapist and a laissez-faire facilitator.* Too, the room was noisy and the chairs uncomfortable. Not exactly an ideal environment or an atmosphere conducive to optimal learning. And proof that we do not choose the spot for our epiphanies.

The first step in EMDR therapy is to have the therapist guide the patient to selecting a target—some troubling aspect of the past or present that the patient wants to rework. A traumatic event—such as a severe accident or the death of a loved one— is a target; so is something ostensibly far less dramatic, like an upsetting memory or a recurrent dream that has replayed in the mind for many years.

The target I chose is known in psychoanalytic terms as a screen memory, something that in and of itself does not seem particularly significant but that, like a dream, disguises deeper, more significant material lying underneath.

In this memory, I must be age four or five. It is afternoon.

My mother is in the hospital, though I don't know why, and I am being looked after not by Mrs. Kenneth, my usual baby-sitter, a kindly elderly women whom I have grown to love and trust, nor by my grandmother, to whom I am attached, but by a strange woman who wears a white uniform with white harlequin glasses and an expression of hostility and disapproval. The grassy area behind our three-story apartment building in Fresh Meadows, Queens, New York, slopes gently upward. She is at the top, and I am at the bottom, innocently wanting to go to a playground nearby. The strange woman is not only hostile to my request but somehow gives me the impression that I am being "bad" for feeling lonely. I am scared of her, vulnerable, and confused. I wish my mother were home.

The memory had remained remarkably vivid in its details, and I described it without faltering. Uri looked at me with his usual analytic contemplation; meanwhile, the unkempt therapist was staring blankly at the manual, attempting to review the instructions.

"What's the negative belief about you that goes with the memory?" he mechanically read aloud. As I'll explain more fully in Chapter 2, *negative cognition* refers to an irrational thought ("I'm worthless," or "I'm stupid") rather than a reality-based one ("It's in the past and I'm safe now"). "It's my fault," I replied.

After the protocol was set (and we will discuss its details in Chapter 2), the therapist began by forgetting the most obvious features of the process. "Aren't you supposed to use hand movements?" Uri asked him. "Isn't the patient supposed to be following those movements with his eyes?"

Yes. The therapist had forgotten. Now the facilitator arrived and demonstrated the correct technique. Between us, Uri and I worked out the hand movements; Uri had to patiently explain to the therapist what his next moves should be and encourage him to keep going. But whatever focus I had mustered was long gone. I remember feeling frustrated, disgusted, resentful, and annoyed.

We began again. Once more I summoned up the target memory, but this time I followed the therapist's hand movement with my eyes. Left right . . . left right . . . left right . . . All of a sudden—*bang!*—a sensation appeared out of nowhere.

I felt something wrapped around my neck! The grip was tightening, and I gasped for air. I was choking!

Quite literally, although I was sitting straight in my chair, I felt my back pinned against a wall. Adrenaline pumped through my system, and my chest was heaving. I was panting as though I had been running for miles. ("Your nostrils were flaring like a racehorse," Uri later told me.)

Except for the terror, the rest was confusion. What or who was choking me? Was this a birth memory of the umbilical cord that almost strangled me? Suddenly I saw a blurry face with expressionless eyes. Was it my sister or the bully next door with hands around my throat? I felt as if I were facing death!

The scene was as vivid as a flashback in a movie; both the sights and the physical sensations were palpable. I was able to be both inside the memory and outside it, participant and observer. For anyone, it would have been a remarkable experience. For me, an experienced therapist, it was mind-blowing.

As the image began to fade, I heard music, faint at first but then growing clearer: Jackson Browne's "Doctor My Eyes."

> Doctor, my eyes
> Cannot see the sky.
> Is this the prize
> For having learned how not to cry?

When the flashback ended, it was immediately followed by another, then another, then another. Five memories in all, each equally vivid, equally powerful.

✳ I'm walking into the high school cafeteria. Two tough kids, far bigger than I, grab me without warning, push me back against a pole, and hold my arms behind it. They say nothing, they are laughing as they try to terrorize me, but I am trapped and helpless. The worst part is that other schoolmates pass by, either not caring or pretending not to see what's happening. It reminds me of not being protected from the bullies I encountered in kindergarten or first grade. Finally I am able to wriggle my arms free and break away. I run over to my usual table and sit down. My friends notice nothing. I am alone. As the memory fades, I quickly jump to another.

✳ I'm in the park with a friend, both of us nine years old. My family has just moved into the neighborhood. (We have moved from Fresh Meadows, a predominantly Jewish middle-class enclave, to Elmhurst, more blue collar, where Jews are a rarity.) Once again, I'm menaced by older, bigger boys who demand to know if I've been baptized. I don't answer, out of defiance more than fear. They hold my friend and me, pinning our arms behind us, and splash filthy puddle water on our heads and faces. I look at one of them squarely in the eye and ask why they have to do this to us. He is briefly taken aback by my trying to reason with him, but moments later they continue splashing us with dirty water. Some adults are in the park and ignore the incident, pretending nothing is happening. The scene ends and abruptly the next begins.

* I'm in my early twenties, traveling by bus along a winding road in Martinique. It's an old, top-heavy bus, and the driver swerves back and forth, right and left, to avoid a wildly driven car. The bus goes out of control. There is absolute silence for what feels like ten seconds, all of us knowing what is about to happen. The bus turns over into a ditch. It is now filled with screams, though not my own. During the split second when my head is catapulted to the metal ceiling, the words *That's it* flash through my mind. I believe I have experienced the final moments of my life. As the image fades into the darkness, the next one pops up.

* I'm nineteen, a camp counselor in Maine. I decide to try snorkeling, so I put on borrowed gear and jump off a dock into the lake water. After enjoying the underwater sights, I surface, believing the tube of the snorkel is out of the water. As I draw in a deep breath, I suck water into my lungs and am immediately seized by exhaustion. Panic grips me. I am suffocating. I grab the water with my weakening arms; twenty feet separate

me from safety. The last few feet are the hardest. Somehow I pull myself up onto the dock and collapse, trying to catch my breath. When at last I can stand, I stagger to the beach, where I lie facedown for what must be half an hour, my head buzzing with the thought that I almost drowned. No one knows nor will ever know unless I tell them. Alone again.

"Time's up," the facilitator interrupted. "We have to switch roles for the next pairing."

I was stunned as I slowly returned to the real world. Uri was looking at me, his expression poker-faced. My therapist, drenched in sweat, was both overwhelmed and amazed. He had been swept along on an unexpected ride through a series of my traumatic memories. The pencil had dropped from his hands, and the manual sat upside down in his lap. Uri reminded us of the last step: the return to the original target.

And then—a miracle! I was barely able to recall the original scene, let alone evoke the emotions it had originally produced. It was as though the nurse baby-sitter never existed; the grief and terror had vanished. The screen was stripped away, and the vivid flashbacks and traumatic memories I'd been carrying for years emerged from the shadows and were freed. Once the memories that were strung along the associated memory pathways had been processed through, the original target unfroze and its emotional power was swept away.

Uri stepped in to handle the final eye movements for me. I saw myself releasing my own hands from my neck. For the first time I realized that throughout my life, I myself had been choking off my life forces, my emotions, creativity, and self-love. As I finished, I heard Bob Marley singing these lines from "Redemption Song":

> Emancipate yourself from mental slavery
> None but ourselves can free our mind.

An hour later, Uri and I left the hotel. We walked in silence, too overwhelmed to speak of what I had undergone. I knew that I had experienced something profound, something transcendent. My first exposure to EMDR had rocked my world, and my mind was racing wildly, jumping from patient to patient, wondering how each of them might respond to this new therapy. I was staggered by the implications of what lay ahead.

How "true" were the flashbacks? Did the remembered incidents really happen?

I was certainly in Martinique on a bus that toppled, I was accosted by boys at my high school, I came within moments of drowning at summer camp, and three kids did "baptize" me with puddle water, to my intense humiliation. But I hadn't consciously realized that I was still traumatized by these events. As for the choking, the most significant flashback: Did it really happen? Could it have been a memory of my difficult birth? Could it possibly have been my older sister choking me? At times during our childhood she let out her jealousy on me. I have a few conscious memories of feeling helpless and controlled when she used her size advantage to pin me to the ground. I also have memories of the boy next door being hostile with me, so I'm just not sure. Memories can be unreliable, and the details were less important to me than the meaning of this flashback.

It took me some days to realize that all the flashbacks had a similar theme: my inability to breathe or to resist being choked while others looked on apathetically. It took me longer still to understand that each flashback was a metaphor for how I remembered aspects of my childhood.

Like all parents, mine carried their life experiences into marriage and child rearing. My father, whose own father was strict and hot-tempered, gained attention in his large family by being well behaved and studious. While his four brothers went into business, he pursued a career in Jewish education, eventually making filmstrips for a variety of Jewish organizations. He was a conscientious objector during World War II and was assigned first as a lumberjack in New Hampshire and then as an orderly in a Connecticut mental hospital. It was tough on me as a kid, when my classmates would boast how their fathers had served in the army or Marines during the war. Somehow, when pressed, I claimed that my father had been in the navy, but I gave no details. Only as an adult could I understand his choice as a powerful act of conscience.

My mother, ten years younger, was more accessible than my dad. She was both vulnerable and resilient. Her father, an affectionate, kind man, was a pharmacist who worked seven days a week to keep his drugstore afloat. Eventually, he saw it flourish, only to have it displaced by the construction of the Triborough

Bridge. His spirit broken, he died of a heart attack when Mom was twenty-one. Her mother was an immaculate housekeeper and cook and, although loving, could be depressed and critical, chasing my mom out of the kitchen with the Yiddish equivalent of "You have clumsy hands." Soon after her husband's death, Mom's mother contracted throat cancer, wasting away at the end in New York Hospital. Soon afterward my mother developed claustrophobia and fears of being unable to breathe. She was anxious about being trapped in a bus or subway and at the movies could only sit in the aisle seat. Hit hard by the death of her parents, she gradually recovered but was haunted by fears of illness and mortality.

My childhood memories of Mom include loving, fun times punctuated by her sadness and fears. I gravitated to the role of emotional caretaker, hating to see her in pain while trying to provide myself with stability. Although full of life and curiosity, I was a shy, insecure child, and by adolescence I was often anxious, underachieving in school and prone to migraine headaches.

My mother had a master's in education, and although she stopped working when my sister was born, she was wonderfully stimulating to my sister's and my creativity. In our younger years, she sat with us at the dining table supervising art projects and storytelling. Although always free with love and affection, my mother struggled with my natural desire to break free.

By contrast, there was much about my father I didn't understand. As I matured, I realized he was a deeply spiritual and emotional man, reserved about his inner life. Dad had high standards, especially with his own brand of morality and scholarship. I rarely heard praise or affection from him, and I grew up uncertain of his love. My mother reassured me that he spoke proudly of me to his friends, but why, I wondered, couldn't he say it to me? When I would playfully drape myself on him, he'd often fend me off with "Don't get too close," and on those rare and thrilling occasions when he played catch with me, he'd quickly lose interest.

My father never realized how much his distance hurt me. Yet I built my own inner bridge to him, identifying with his perseverance and innovative qualities. I have followed in his footsteps by becoming a writer and lecturer.

My relationship with my sister raised the most confusion of all. She was three years older, and we shared the same room until I was nine. She could be a bright and creative playmate; eventually she opened to me the world of rock and roll and dating. But she alternated between being loving and being hurtful. Her occasional bouts of jealousy led her to use her size and sophistication to her advantage. (It wasn't entirely one-sided; I had the usual rivalrous feelings toward her.) My best defense against her was to be the easier child for my parents, my way of retaliating. But I rarely knew what I had done to warrant her resentment.

Early on I devised ways of suppressing painful thoughts and feelings. By midadolescence, most of my positive feelings were frozen along with the negative ones I was containing. My self-choking had reached full force. As a result, my maturity level slipped behind that of many of my peers. I floated through Queens College aimlessly, continuing my pattern of academic underachievement. I dated occasionally and had my first major relationship with a girl—four years my junior. I experimented with marijuana—for me, a step toward independence and normalcy—and remember walking into the student union to play Pong, high on pot, as Eric Clapton's *Crossroads* blared on the speakers.

The Vietnam War was in full swing. My father encouraged me to register as a conscientious objector. I was afraid to disappoint him and I was against the war, but I was no pacifist, and when I came to the question, "Are you against all wars in any form?" on the registration form, I answered no to the question and made myself eligible.

I had a student deferment, however, and in my senior year, President Nixon ended the draft. I was driving down to Philadelphia when I heard the news on the car radio, and I had to pull over to absorb the news. I was safe, knowing that hundreds of thousands of other guys weren't that fortunate, shipped back home in body bags, on crutches, and with tormented souls. Decades later I was honored by the opportunity to help heal their traumas with EMDR.

Decisions had to be made about my future course and my choice of graduate studies. My own search for inner meaning led me to think about becoming a psychotherapist. Getting into a doctoral program in psychology required an A average, which I didn't have. So I applied to and was accepted by Yeshiva University School of Social Work in its master's program, an alternative route into the psychotherapy field. I enjoyed the classes, but trouble brewed in my field placement, a hospital mental health clinic. I started my day at the clinic at 9:00 A.M., and like clockwork, by two o'clock every afternoon, I developed a kick-in-the-stomach abdominal pain. My suppressed emotions were demanding attention. My supervisor picked up problems in my work with clients, about which I was clueless. It got so bad that she passed me that first semester only on the condition that I enter therapy.

Within two weeks of starting therapy, as I started a process of self-exploration and healing that continues to this day, my stomachaches disappeared. I graduated with highest honors. I got my first paying job (at a princely $12,700 a year) as a social worker at a vocational rehabilitation agency and rented a studio apartment in Queens. At work the lunatic behavior came more from the administrators than from the emotionally disturbed patients, but it was a trial by fire, from which I learned a tremendous amount about working with shattered people. The staff social workers bonded together for mutual support and learning. One of them was Nina Cohen, who entranced me with her beauty, sweetness, and wisdom. Three years later I took a position as a senior social worker (later clinical director) in a counseling center on Long Island. Nina and I married, moved to a town house in the suburbs, and had a child, Jonathan, who remains a blessing to us both. I have no trouble setting limits for him—or in telling him, daily, how much I love him, but parenthood is still parenthood, with all its ups and downs.

In 1981 I started a part-time practice, and a year later I left the clinic to become a full-time private therapist. I was accepted into a psychoanalytic training institute that entailed three years of study and a personal analysis. It laid the cornerstone for my knowledge of how to understand and help with the complex challenges presented by those seeking my help.

For seventeen years I continued to study. I earned a more-than-adequate living and considered myself content if not particularly fulfilled. I was able to feel emotion, to experience and express pleasure and joy, to relate to friends, acquaintances, and strangers, and even to speak in public and walk confidently into a cocktail party.

I was, in short, ready for something remarkable. I was ready for EMDR.

Age forty may seem late to find one's calling, but the world is full of people who realized their potential in their thirties or in middle age. (Thomas Mann, for example, did not write his first novel until he was thirty-nine.) Perhaps I wasn't ready to expand until I had learned to face my emotions rather than try to escape them, a process that had taken all those years. Perhaps I simply had to meet and be inspired by Francine Shapiro.

In any event, thanks to EMDR I changed from a person who was a successful psychotherapist on Long Island to one who has succeeded internationally, from a boy who was reluctant to leave home to a man who has gone to Belfast to help its citizens recover from twenty-five years of The Troubles. EMDR has enabled me to treat victims of severe trauma, witnesses to and victims of devastation from train wrecks to the dangerous streets of Bedford-Stuyvesant. I have helped dramatically improve the performance of professional athletes and creative artists, including developing a unique acting method incorporating EMDR technology. Along with others, I have built on Francine Shapiro's foundation with innovative ways of making EMDR even more effective, with a wider application to life's challenges. In this book, I'll describe some of my most dramatic encounters, take you to the heights that EMDR can reach, and prove that traumas don't have to produce lifelong scars—indeed, can be healed—*sometimes within hours!* (In many cases of profound childhood trauma, however, healing with EMDR can, as we'll see, take many months or a number of years.)

In the course of my journey and in my practice, especially since learning EMDR, I've learned many truths that transcend any therapeutic technique or belief system.

- It is therapeutic for therapists to be open and comfortable with the fact that, like those who seek their help, they are vulnerable and flawed. It is antitherapeutic for therapists to hide behind their superior position in the power relationship.
- Therapy works best when two people find their way together, one needing help with a problem, the other being able to act as a guide in problem solving, but in all other respects being equal.
- The good therapist gives the patient experience of another person as well as the experience of the patient himself.
- The therapist who does not learn from her patient is not doing her job fully.

- The brain has the capacity to heal from intractable memories, emotions, and beliefs just as the body can heal from physical injury. It will do so spontaneously, when the obstacles to healing are removed.

- The only meaningful answers lie within the patient's mind, body, and spirit. Therapists can never *on their own* come close to understanding what a patient's core issues are—we're always off. Optimal therapy guides a patient to find answers from within and to make use of them, without outside influence from the therapist.

- We do not have to accept being "stuck for life" with painful symptoms, poor self-images, or negative tapes that spin endlessly in our minds. "Miracle" change, once thought impossible, is now possible, sometimes at warp speed!

Given these universal truths, the right method—at least EMDR—is greater than any particular therapist. All therapists who use it can benefit their patients. All who "take" it can be helped.

But what precisely *is* EMDR? How has it changed and expanded? Why am I so convinced of its efficacy?

The best way to answer these questions is to take you through the background of EMDR: its development, theory, and practice. Then I will share with you my own experience, from an awed and deeply moved recipient to a seasoned practitioner. After that, I will show it to you—and show you myself—in action.

CHAPTER 2
CHAPTER 2
CHAPTER 2
CHAPTER 2
CHAPTER 2
CHAPTER 2
CHAPTER 2
CHAPTER 2 **THE THEORY OF EMDR**

The fact that eye movements from left to right, right to left, have physiological and psychological effects has been known for a long time. Hypnotists at times use these movements as an aid in inducing a trance state. The controversial psychiatrist Wilhelm Reich postulated that "loosening" the eyes was a path toward releasing unexpressed emotions and feelings. The act of reading itself deepens understanding of what is being read. People rapt in thought will move their eyes without realizing it.

Indeed, any bilateral movement, not just eye movement, affects the brain, in some cases stimulating it, in others relaxing it or freeing it from anxiety and stress. African drums, depending on their cadence, can excite an audience or calm it. Sound has far greater effect when experienced stereophonically than monaurally. Long-distance runners, whose legs move in a regular rhythm, speak both of entering a "zone" and of their heightened ability for problem solving. Bilateral stimulation tends to bring out what's uppermost in your mind and then help you let it go, leading to a relaxation response.

It was Francine Shapiro's genius to see how this phenomenon could be applied therapeutically.

THE ORIGINS

"The seed of EMDR sprouted one sunny afternoon in 1987, when I took a break to ramble around a small lake," writes Dr. Shapiro in her 1997 book, *EMDR: The Breakthrough "Eye Movement" Therapy for Overcoming Anxiety, Stress, and Trauma.* "I noticed that when a disturbing thought entered my mind, my eyes spontaneously started moving back and forth. They were making rapid movements on a diagonal from lower left to upper right. At the same time, I noticed that my disturbing thought had shifted from consciousness, and when I brought it back to mind, it no longer bothered me as much" (p. 9).

She tried it again, this time deliberately, picking out an anxiety-producing thought and moving her eyes. The result was the same. She tried it with friends and acquaintances. Again the process worked, though she often had to guide their eye movements by having them follow her finger. But while their anxiety lessened, it did not altogether disappear, and she realized she had to develop a procedure to resolve the anxiety more thoroughly. "I learned," she explains, "that I had to ask the person to change the focus of his attention (to a different aspect of the thing he was upset about) or lead his eyes in a different way, perhaps horizontally, or faster, or slower. The more I experimented, the more I found the need to come up with alternatives to jump-start the positive effect when it became stalled."

Thus was born the key concept of a *target* or a succession of targets, depending on the length of the therapy. But before I describe them and how they are used in the therapeutic protocol, it's important to understand just a little about the brain.

LEFT BRAIN, RIGHT BRAIN

You've surely read about the two sides of the brain, the right governing emotion and creativity, the left cognitive thinking. This delineation is oversimplified, even simplistic, for there is continuous interaction between all parts of the brain. The brain's wiring is an endlessly complex system of neurons and synapses; there are more than four *quadrillion* connections that we now understand in only the most limited of ways.

The brain is an incredibly complex system made up of a variety of structures, many of which lie in both the left and the right hemispheres. But the brain is also divided into three other segments: the human brain, the mammalian brain, and the reptilian brain. The human brain is also known as the forebrain, the thinking or cortical brain; the mammalian brain is also known as the midbrain, the emotional or limbic brain; the reptilian brain, at the base of the skull, is also known as the hindbrain or the primitive brain, governing autonomic functions such as REM sleep, reflex, circulation, and respiration. The lower hindbrain, the brainstem, connects with the rest of the nervous system at the top of the spinal column. This is the true mind-body connection, since all information traveling from the brain to the body and back passes through this portal.

Despite the attention given to the mechanisms of the brain in recent decades, top experts in neurology admit that they still know little about its workings. Our understanding of how EMDR works is accordingly quite limited. Many theories have been proposed, the simplest being that alternating bilateral stimulation enhances communication between the left and the right brains. In this theory, the rapid, powerful flow of EMDR processing intensifies the constant communication of all the interconnected brain structures. The parallels between the eye movements in EMDR and those in REM sleep are obvious, as is the information processing that goes on during both activities. Robert Stickgold, Ph.D., a neurology researcher at Harvard University, has speculated that the flow of information from the hippocampus (which stores information) to the neocortex (which analyzes information) is directionally reversed in EMDR, as is the case during REM cycles, allowing the brain to reevaluate information frozen in a system that was overwhelmed at the time of the traumatic event. Others believe that EMDR works because its alternating distraction effect activates a continuous startle response, unsettling the brain and causing an unsettling and reworking of dysfunctionally stored information. Both these ideas make sense and are likely pieces of a much larger puzzle that we are just beginning to assemble.

THE COURSE OF EMDR THERAPY

THE FIRST STEPS

A therapist, of course, has much work to do with a patient before the actual bilateral stimulation and complex brain activation begin. Typically, during their initial meeting, the therapist will take a history of the patient. This basic step in all doctor-patient relationships is particularly important here because the EMDR therapist knows how powerful a patient's response to EMDR can be and wants to make sure that it will not be overwhelming. EMDR is most immediately helpful to moderately traumatized, anxious, or stressed people; it can be dangerously disruptive for the severely disturbed, with whom the therapist must proceed cautiously and slowly.

After the history is taken, the therapist explains how the process works and what to expect. The client is informed that a less complex issue, such as a single traumatic incident in adulthood (a car accident or a mugging), may be resolved in a few sessions, but that a more complex problem, which usually results from a history of childhood trauma and abuse, is deeply ingrained in the system and may take months or even years of ongoing EMDR treatment to fully heal. A client who is presenting a discrete trauma is informed that forgotten traumas from earlier in life may emerge and complicate and lengthen the treatment process.

IDENTIFYING THE TARGET

The therapist then asks the patient to select a target—a troubling incident, memory, or image, or even a particular feeling, such as panic or sadness. For the therapist, it's easier to work with a specific event. If the complaint is more general ("I suffer from panic attacks"), then the therapist must try to track down the source of the feeling. "When was the first time you experienced this panic?" he or she will ask. "What was going on in your life at the time?" One of Francine Shapiro's most effective approaches was to ask the patient three questions: When was the earliest time you had the feeling? When was the worst time? When was the most recent time? Ultimately, all three responses can be used as targets, but we generally start with the most powerful ("the worst time"). Still, the therapist must be careful not to lead the client. EMDR is patient-centered, and it is the therapist's job to guide the patient to choose and formulate his or her own target. Unlike other forms of therapy, EMDR does not work on assumption. A target is designated, and the patient is guided to visualize the worst or most resonant moment of the memory. (The *image* activates the aspect of the memory held in the occipital cortex, which controls sight in the brain.) The client is also asked if any sounds or smells arise with the visual memories.

IDENTIFYING THE NEGATIVE COGNITION

The next step is to elicit the *negative cognition* associated with the designated image. A rape victim's belief that it was her fault, or that she is "dirty," is a good example, for these are both distortions, *irrational* beliefs; irrationality is the cornerstone of negative cognition. These beliefs are the "thinking symptoms" of the trauma. "I shouldn't have walked in the park after midnight," for example, is a *rational* belief and thus is not a negative cognition in the sense that we use that term.

The therapist's art lies in bringing out what the client really believes, not what he *thinks* is an appropriate belief, and to help the client find the best words to express it. A particular therapist might never associate a client's negative thought with the target, but if the client does, then the thought is "right." For instance, if a patient has been rear-ended in a car accident, one might expect him to say—irrationally, since it was he who was rear-ended—"It's my fault we crashed." But if instead he says, "I'm a totally incompetent person," it might be surprising, but it is the patient's true negative cognition, and the therapist should not alter it.

It should, however, be released, for this is the purpose of EMDR therapy. The rational brain knows what is distorted and what is not, and EMDR allows the patient to see the distortion and replace it with something more accurate. "I'm afraid now when I drive" is a reasonable emotion; the patient doesn't want to get hit again. But "I'm destined to have an accident every time I drive" and "Terrible things always happen to me" are distorted feelings, and it is EMDR's triumph that it allows the patient to let them go.

The therapist needs to educate the client as to what a negative cognition is and then help him or her find it. The therapist does not put words in the client's mouth, but instead guides her to express her innermost thoughts or convictions. The target and its symptoms are neurologically entwined, coming from various regions of the patient's brain. The initial targeting is an effort to "light up" the part(s) of the brain where the image or memory is "stuck." The bilateral stimulation will act as a kind of cerebral pacemaker, activating and moving thought. Scientists know from brain scans that depression, anxiety, panic, and trauma correlate with increased blood flow on the right side of the brain. As trauma and its symptoms heal, the scans show, activity balances more equally for both sides of the brain.

Ultimately, EMDR normalizes activity. Through bilateral stimulation, the unprocessed memory or image does not remain frozen in state but proceeds from being a traumatic memory (feeling as if it just happened, is happening, or is going to happen) to being a memory experienced as from the past. And once it's released, the patient will never go back and reactivate the same image or its emotional charge.

Ted's Negative Cognition

Ted, a man of forty, comes into my office in a depressed state. A successful salesman (patients' names and identities have been disguised), he dresses well and keeps himself in good shape. Yet he has not been able to hold his marriage together, and now he finds himself constantly anxious that he will fumble away his job as well. He is, he tells me, the younger of two sons and has always felt that his parents preferred his brother.

I explain the concept of a target and ask him to choose one.

"My brother used to beat me up all the time," he tells me.

This is a good beginning, but more is needed. "When did it start?" I ask him.

"As far back as I can remember."

"When was the most recent time?"

"Twenty years ago, before he went off to college."

"When was the worst time?"

He pauses for a moment. "I was fifteen, he was eighteen. He hit me so hard he broke my tooth."

"Can you see that image?"

"I do," he says, but the response is unnecessary. I can tell by the way his eyes light up and the sudden defensive slouch in his posture that he can see it.

"I can taste the blood and feel the pain in my mouth, also," he added.

"When you see that picture, what negative, distorted, self-critical, irrational thought comes to mind?" I am asking about the negative cognition. "Something you're still carrying, even if you know it isn't true. And remember: It isn't what you thought then, it's what comes to you now."

He answers without hesitation. "I'm weak."

His build belies his words. I could contradict him, but that would be a therapeutic mistake. "I'm weak" has psychological and physical implications. If he had said, "I *was* weak," then it would have been a statement of fact, inappropriate for our use.

"Is that true?" I ask him to provide further validation.

He reconsiders. "Uh . . . no."

His contradiction comes too quickly. It appears that he can go deeper. "If it's not that, what would be more like it?"

"I'm sad."

While in some cases, this might be a distorted, negative belief to the speaker, in Ted's case it's obviously true. He *is* sad.

I probe further. "What makes you sad?"

"Nobody loves me. And they're right. I'm worthless."

We have reached Ted's most profound *negative cognition*—as well as a stopping place in his story. It's time to discuss the next step in the protocol.

FINDING THE POSITIVE COGNITION

Once a negative cognition has been elicited, the next step is to give the client something to shoot for—something positive, affirming. This is a way of activating semantic areas in the left prefrontal lobe—that is, of lighting up an optimistic area of the brain.

The *positive cognition* needn't be the direct opposite of the negative cognition. "I'm strong" is not an antidote to "I'm weak," nor is "I'm great" the likely positive cognition stemming from "I'm worthless." A positive cognition must be a thought that the patient can fully perceive as realistic in the now. The brain has to be able to take it in, acknowledge that it is accurate, *and believe it.* For Ted, "I can handle myself now" might be an appropriate positive cognition, for it is a considered, rational belief. But again the positive cognition must be the patient's *own*; the therapist must refrain from imposing her own words.

USING RATING SCALES

Now we come to EMDR's most defining therapeutic task. Once we have identified negative and positive cognitions, we must tangibly determine their depth and power. This rating process is done (no surprise!) by the client, but the therapist can play a direct part in eliciting the answers by using rating scales.

Two different scales are used. The Validity of Cognition (VOC) scale, developed by Francine Shapiro, is applied to the positive cognition. It simply asks the patient, "How true does your positive cognition feel right now when you pair it with the target image?" The rating is done numerically, on a scale of 1 to 7, with 1 meaning "totally false" and 7 denoting "totally true." Ted rated his positive cognition that he could handle himself as a two—almost completely false.

The other scale, developed by the behavioral psychologist Joseph Wolpe, is called the Subjective Unit of Disturbance Scale (SUDS). It asks the patient to pair the target image with the negative cognition and then observe whatever feelings are elicited. The therapist need not understand why a particular image and negative cognition generate the emotions they do, nor believe that the emotions are appropriate to the trauma. Again, the negative cognition belongs to the client, and if he feels it, then SUDS is applicable to it. The emotions associated with the cognition can be fear, sadness, envy, panic, even joy— whatever spontaneously comes up.

The therapist using SUDS then asks, "On a scale of zero

to ten, if you were to rate how distressing the emotions feel right at this moment, where ten represents the worst you could feel and zero represents neutral, what number goes along with the feelings?" I am continually surprised at how quickly the responses come: "Six." "Nine." "Five and a half." The answers are often given with expressions and postures that mirror the emotions; if the emotion is sadness, tears often flow.

The purpose of EMDR is to bring the SUDS down to 0 and then raise the VOC up to 7. Sometimes, even in the case of severe trauma, this can be accomplished *in a single session*! This is why "warp speed" is part of this book's title.

Before the therapist starts the bilateral stimulation, one more question needs to be answered: "Where in your body do you feel the distress now?" If the patient has difficulty locating the sensations, the therapist guides the patient to scan the body from head to toe. It is a testament to the mind/body connection that emotions are almost always expressed in body sensations. Again, it isn't of importance for the therapist to understand the meaning of the response (a patient of mine once answered, "Over the top of my head"), but it is necessary for the patient to physically locate the feeling, activating the most deeply held emotions. For the EMDR process to be completed, the body has to be cleared of all distress.

Just before the left-right stimulation begins, the therapist explains that as the process goes on, the patient's mind is going to move. Do not try to direct it, the therapist explains; simply let it flow. As Dr. Shapiro teaches, it's like gazing out a train window, seeing what goes by. You simply observe.

BILATERAL STIMULATION

Three modes are used to activate bilaterality: alternating eye movements, tactile stimulation (touch), and auditory stimulation (sound). With eye movements, the eyes generally move horizontally, left to right, right to left, tracking the therapist's fingers. With tactile stimulation, the therapist taps or presses first one hand of the patient, then the other, in a steady rhythm. With auditory stimulation, the patient dons headsets and listens to sound that alternately flows into one ear and then the other. These are the most common methods of bilateral stimulation, and while Francine Shapiro started with eye movements, they all are effective, although people have their individual preferences. (The advantage to touch and sound, the more passive approaches, over eye movements is that, unless patients get overwhelmed, they can close their eyes and focus internally on their images.) I have used all three methods, both separately and in combination, depending on what I deemed most appropriate. All work.

The patient has been told to let the process flow. (In my own first session, as I've said, images—entire scenes—rapidly played out in my mind, some of them accompanied by music and lyrics, one after another.) The information processing stage of EMDR then begins. During sets of bilateral stimulation, without conscious effort, the patient's attention shifts from the target image to the negative cognition, the emotions it evokes, and the place in the body that houses the emotions, as an organic whole. The patient goes inward, observing without speaking, often crying or laughing, invariably profoundly moved. Talking to the therapist takes place only between sets, when the patient can relate as much or as little of her experience as she chooses. Movement and resolution occur internally, independent of the therapist's awareness. The process belongs to the patient. After reflecting her experience, she is encouraged to continue, guided by the therapist to "go with that."

The process can last as long as three hours, or as little as thirty minutes, depending on the scheduled length of the session and the amount of material that comes up. Only when the patient appears to be approaching the point of resolution does the therapist bring her back to the target, in order to assess the progress and the current level of distress. This is accomplished by directing the patient to reaccess the original image, which oftentimes has changed in clarity or perspective, and (using SUDS) to rate the level of distress by pairing it with the original negative cognition. When the number comes up as a 0 or 1, the process is finished, or close to it. If the number is higher, the ongoing work resumes from the current state of the target.

When the stress has evaporated, the time has arrived to install the positive cognition, which the brain is now ready to accept and strengthen. The VOC is obtained by pairing the original target image with the positive cognition. The rating is invariably higher and at times is near or at 7. The positive cognition is now installed with the same bilateral stimulation that has been used up to this juncture, until it feels firmly true.

Two elements are at work here:

✳ Complete and permanent desensitization of a traumatic memory or a distressing feeling or belief (rare in other forms of psychotherapy), which takes away the distress level of the original target.

✳ Processing in, or deepening, the positive cognition, meaning that the negative, distorted belief will be replaced by a positive, realistic belief. (After this work, Ted felt he was capable of handling attacks similar to the ones meted out by his brother.)

When the process is complete, the brain has discarded the distorted, subjective experience that had overwhelmed and remained frozen in the patient and replaced it with a positive perception of present reality. Technically, the EMDR process links up disparate or unconnected neural networks, which connects them to reality, and new, accurate information is allowed to flow through to the patient's consciousness along paths that were heretofore blocked.

Like the body's immune system, the neurophysiological system recovers when obstacles to its healing are removed. Our brain protects us, keeps us in balance. Trauma disrupts this process. A flashback, a startling reliving of an overwhelming experience, reveals unprocessed information that is frozen in the nervous system. EMDR is the means of reaching *and reactivating* the area (or areas) where the trauma is trapped. Bilateral stimulation drives the linking of that targeted trauma to other parts of the brain and in so doing releases the trauma. But it is not the bilateral stimulation alone that effects the cure—it is the entire process. That is the ultimate miracle of EMDR.

DR. SHAPIRO'S ONGOING CONTRIBUTIONS

It has been fourteen years since Francine Shapiro took her walk around the lake. Thanks initially to her teaching, vision, and determination—and her ability to weather reflexive derision of the scientific and academic communities—but thanks ultimately to its own effectiveness, EMDR is now practiced around the world. For the first five years, Dr. Shapiro personally conducted every training session here and abroad, stressing the importance of diligently following her protocols and procedures. At present 40,000 therapists have trained with the EMDR Institute, and new generations of practitioners are integrating her powerful method with new techniques and applications. I have introduced the use of bilateral music and nature sounds, which can be used continuously through sessions instead of the interrupted sets of eye movements. And I have initiated protocols tailored especially for performance, creativity, and acting. Some see my stretching of the boundaries as heresy, others as inspiration.

Discovering and developing a treatment method that is revolutionizing the mental health field worldwide has not been enough for Francine Shapiro. A true visionary, she soon recognized that the power of EMDR to rapidly heal trauma had humanitarian implications. She observed how the cycle of violence potentially turns some of today's victims into tomorrow's perpetrators—and saw that healing could break that cycle. She recognized that, for both economic and social reasons, those who needed this help the most tended to receive it least.

With the help of other EMDR pioneers, she developed EMDR Humanitarian Assistance Programs (HAP), which has provided pro bono training and treatment at disaster sites (in Oklahoma City after the bombing of the federal building and in Homestead, Florida, after Hurricane Andrew) and in areas of suffering around the world (Bosnia, Rwanda, Central and South America). It has also provided healing for Vietnam and other combat veterans.

Dr. Shapiro's inspiration and mentorship guided me to organize humanitarian trainings in Northern Ireland as well as in Bedford-Stuyvesant, an inner-city community in Brooklyn. These were peak experiences for me, and along with my receiving and providing EMDR therapy, they have opened me up and altered the course of my life in ways I never could have imagined.

EMDR has helped me. It lets me help others. And from the beginning Francine Shapiro's discovery convinced me that "miracles" are possible.

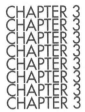
CHAPTER 3
CHAPTER 3
CHAPTER 3
CHAPTER 3
CHAPTER 3
CHAPTER 3
CHAPTER 3

CHAPTER 3 MY APPRENTICESHIP

In the beginning, my transition into becoming an EMDR practitioner wasn't exactly smooth. One intense training weekend, one that gave me a mind-blowing personal encounter with EMDR, did not fully prepare me for its use. On the first day after that weekend, I went back to my office, curious to try out this new methodology with my patients. I knew the protocol, I had experienced the effects. Now it was time to put the method into practice.

PHILIP: THE LAWYER

I had eight patients scheduled for that day, and I decided to use EMDR with three of them as trauma appeared to block their progress. The first, Philip, a man in his early forties, was an associate attorney with whom I had been working for one and a half years. He was a mild-mannered, somewhat obsessive person, in need of constant praise and encouragement, and given to bouts of anxiety and depression, especially whenever he was criticized. Through medication and therapy he had progressed; he now understood that an overbearing father in his childhood lay behind his adult fears and passivity. Still, his depression lingered in a milder form, and the prospect of confrontation still sent him spiraling.

I explained that I had learned a new therapeutic technique and asked if he wanted to try it out. He agreed so readily, I was concerned that he might be overriding possible inner objections. Since I was embarking on something entirely new, I followed Francine Shapiro's guidelines word for word. I asked him what memory he wanted to target.

"A meeting last week with one of the partners," he told me. "He wanted me to inflate a client's account, and when I refused, he loomed over me like the wrath of God. Of course what he was asking was illegal, but that didn't matter to him. He accused me of not being a team player." Philip paused, his breathing rapid and his face beet red. "Even if I challenge him mildly, he's all over me. He tells me I don't have the stuff, that I shouldn't have become a lawyer in the first place, that I'll never make partner. And it's not fair. It's *just not fair!*" His head bowed; he could not continue.

"Can you hear his voice now?" I asked.

"Oh, yeah."

"What's the negative belief that accompanies the image and the sound of his voice?"

His answer was immediate. "It's true. I'm incompetent."

"What emotions go with the image and the negative belief?"

"Anxiety, guilt, shame."

"Where do you feel it in your body?"

"My stomach is churning."

With Philip fully activated, I began moving my hand—twenty-four movements to the right and to the left, the baseline Francine had recommended. His mind started to race. He remembered other incidents when he felt bullied by the partners in his firm, then incidents when he had been verbally attacked by his father. As he went on, I was aware that I was making some technical mistakes, but I did not interrupt him—the images were coming too fast for us to stop. When he finally grew quiet, I took him back to the original image.

"It's gone," he said.

Despite all I had learned just the previous day, I was incredulous.

"Gone?"

"Yes. I can't bring it up."

"And the negative belief?"

"It just doesn't make sense now. I'm not incompetent. I'm one of the best lawyers in the firm!"

He shook his head in wonder at his own words.

"And how does your body feel?"

"Relaxed."

"Your stomach?"

"Peaceful."

Immediately after he left, I mentally replayed what had just happened. Of one thing I was sure: This bore no resemblance to anything that I had ever run into before as a therapist. The speed with which Philip had changed, and the degree of his transformation, left me dumbfounded. I had access to a new and powerful system, and its effects seemed too good to be true.

POLLY: THE STUDENT

The results with my second patient, though not quite as spectacular, increased my amazement. Polly was a twenty-year-old college student with a round, pleasant face, dark hair, and eyes that seemed to look at the world in perpetual wonder. She was entangled in a self-defeating relationship with a young man—what was, for her, a familiar situation. During the few months she had been coming to me, she had dubbed herself as a "serial masochist," as she couldn't break free from this man who, she was certain, was unfaithful to her.

She chose a recent memory, and the image came to her in a flash. She was on the telephone with her boyfriend, having waited for his call all day, and now he was telling her "something had come up" and he couldn't see her. She was sure it was because he was seeing someone else, and as she hung up, she felt intense shame and degradation.

"What negative belief goes with that image?" I asked.

"I don't deserve anything good."

"Your emotions?"

"Guilt, shame."

"Distress level?"

"Ten."

"What do you feel in your body?"

"A sinking feeling in my stomach."

Again, I used the prescribed number of eye movements, but I felt like a juggler who was becoming adept at keeping three balls in the air and suddenly had to handle eight. Images, activated by the EMDR, flashed through Polly's mind. A girlfriend teasing her when she was seven. Her big brother playing doctor with her when she was ten. She couldn't repeat everything that was going on in her head, and in previous therapy we would have focused on only one situation, not a slew of them. Here I did not interrupt the flow of images. It was a virgin experience for her and the second for me, and each of us was bewildered by the rapidity of the process. Nevertheless, when I brought her back to her original image, she reported that it had "faded," that her negative belief seemed "disconnected" from it, less painful and more dispassionate, and that her body felt relaxed.

When Polly left, I was again bewildered. Philip's image had disappeared, hers had faded. Still, the notion that I could resolve a painful memory to the point where there was no distress in so short a time was as alien to me as intergalactic travel.

MAGGIE: THE ACTRESS

Perhaps in response to my confusion, I waited until my last patient of the day before using EMDR again. Maggie, at thirty-eight, was a voluble actress, skilled in putting on a good front;

she worked in sales to support herself in her acting career. Despite her creative gifts and an uncanny ability to slip into any character, she had undermined her own efforts to attain theatrical success; her brave face masked a history of disappointments. She, like Polly, had suffered through a string of destructive relationships, and though we had been working together for five years, tangible results were still scarce. Maggie hid behind protective armor (which therapists see as a powerful narcissistic defense), and I even wondered why she kept coming to see me. If it weren't for her perseverance and my own stubborn unwillingness to give up on a person—I hate to turn away anyone who is trying—I might have raised the possibility of referring her to another therapist. But I realized that a deep wound lay hidden underneath her exterior. Her father had hit her when she was a child, her mother was often sick and inaccessible, and Maggie herself suffered from depression and panic attacks. Knowing this, I couldn't turn her away. But even after five years, I was unable to gauge the extent of the trauma that afflicted her.

Today Maggie seemed unusually nervous. (Had she picked up on my own uncertainty?) Her voice was constricted as she agreed to the new therapeutic technique, and when I began my questioning, she stared at me almost challengingly.

The target image that came to her was of her oldest sister (she had three altogether) pushing her down on the bed and not letting her get up.

"What's your negative belief?"

"I'm helpless." Her voice became that of a little girl. "I *am* totally helpless."

The statement "I'm helpless" is different from the more common "I'm worthless," revealing not a self-attack but a loss of control. It was the first time in all those years that I had made contact with the genuine Maggie, the inside Maggie. We hadn't used eye movement yet, but she was already emerging. Panic, she said, was rising in her chest.

"On a scale of zero to ten, what is your distress level?" I asked.

"A nine," she said, although from the hint of terror in her eyes, I would have judged it off the scale.

Then we started. She careened through memories of her helplessness, with her parents, onstage, with her sisters; there were many images of childhood verbal and physical abuse. Her mind worked at warp speed until all was calm. I directed her back to her original image. The amount of time that had passed could not have been more than ten minutes.

"It disappeared," she said.

It's impossible, not this quickly, I thought, but simply asked her about her distress level.

"Zero," she reflected matter-of-factly.

No way! I pushed and probed, convinced that her symptoms were playing hide-and-seek, trying to make some sense of what appeared to be a therapeutic miracle. (Five years of crawling, and now, after ten minutes using EMDR, a breakthrough!)

I asked Maggie once more about her sisters, about the scene on the bed. This time there was neither defensiveness nor childlike vulnerability. She was present and composed; we talked as though we were discussing the weather.

I was literally stunned. I could not think rationally. My brain locked on the only possible explanation:

The three patients set me up! They consulted each other on the phone—they acted in collusion!

Absurd as the idea was, for a brief period I couldn't shake it. But of course in reality Philip, Polly, and Maggie did not know each other, and even if they had, they would not have concocted this preposterous scheme. No, I was getting a crash course in the power of EMDR.

When Maggie came back the next week, she did not mention what had transpired, even though her anxiety was gone. We had a rich and profound therapeutic session. I itched to ask her about our last session, and at last I could contain myself no longer. Her answer let me see that on the one hand, the change in her was profound, but on the other that—like a wound that is healed and no longer hurts—it was difficult to recognize that shift.

"Would you like to do more EMDR," I suggested.

She looked at me in mild surprise. "Oh," she said, waving her hand back and forth, "that silly thing?"

You would think that after the miraculous results on the first day, I would have started to use the technique all the time, but a variety of factors held me back. I still couldn't explain EMDR's power, which left me anxious and confused. My own patients minimized the impact of EMDR. And I had no colleagues besides Uri with whom to discuss my cases either theoretically or technically. Under these circumstances I held back. When I did use EMDR, I found myself straying from its protocols and mistrustful of its effects. It was a valuable thera-

peutic tool, I decided, but it was too alien to me and to everything I had been taught.

Six months later I took Level II training, but even this was
not enough to propel me, fully committed, into consistently
using EMDR. Ironically, despite the dramatic changes my
clients experienced, very few of them would come to sessions
and ask for the treatment. They were picking up on my lack of
confidence and not realizing the nature and significance of
their own organic shifts. Although I was in danger of becoming an EMDR dropout, somehow I persevered, even if I was
limping along.

Fortunately my good friend Uri, accompanied by another
friend and colleague, Mark Dworkin—also a Long Island
EMDR therapist—told me they were going out to Los Angeles to be trained as EMDR facilitators—those who teach the
method hands on in the practicum section of the trainings.
They asked if I wanted to join them, and I hesitated. *Why
should I learn to teach others if I'm not sure of it myself?* I thought.
"This is your last opportunity—they're closing the list for facilitators in New York State," Mark told me. I decided to go for it.
Good choice.

So in January 1995, eighteen months after I had taken my
Level I training, I flew out to Los Angeles for facilitator training with Uri and Mark. The night before the session started, we
acted like teenagers in our hotel suite, releasing tension with
physical pranks and put-down humor.

On the brink of training to become a facilitator, I thought
back to how overwhelming my first experience had been and

sensed the heavy responsibility of taking on the role of teacher. At the Los Angeles training, there were a number of advanced EMDR facilitators who would act as our teachers, oversee our work, and let us treat them with EMDR to observe our skills. They were all top-notch.

Francine Shapiro was there, too.

In my earlier trainings, I had marveled at her brilliance, her capacity for clarity, and the inspirational tenor of her remarks. The method was new to me, and although I was astounded by my own response to it, I had integrated only bits and pieces of what she had said.

This time was different. This time I really got it. When she lectured, it was as if her words flowed directly into my brain. What I understood now was what Francine had discovered in her walk around the lake: the basic components of the therapy, how they fit together, and how they work. I took in the profound simplicity that had contributed to this profound shift in our understanding of the human mind and the healing of its traumas.

This understanding would deepen and expand in the years to come, enabling me to contribute my own interpretations, my own techniques, to what Francine had pioneered. But in that Los Angeles session, I felt filled with inspiration. The power of EMDR seemed no longer a mystery (and certainly not intimidating) but rather a therapeutic tool far more potent than any I had ever encountered—and I gained new confidence in my ability to master it.

When I returned home, I began using EMDR with all my new patients, and I gradually integrated it into the treatment of my ongoing patients. Two months after the Los Angeles trip, I facilitated at one of Dr. Shapiro's Level II trainings, and my learning curve skyrocketed further. It hit me that I did not have to discard the theories and techniques I had succeeded with for years. I could integrate EMDR with a psychodynamic approach to therapy. Dr. Shapiro had inspired me not only with her ideas but with her ability to integrate existing wisdom and create something new.

RALPH: THE PAINTER

A few weeks later I treated my first discrete trauma case. Ralph was a soft-spoken man of thirty-six, blue-eyed and burly with light blond hair. A house painter, he had been working in the cellar of a suburban residential home when a frayed electrical wire set fire to nearby cans of turpentine. Within seconds flames consumed the room, and only because he had the good luck to be standing near the sole window was Ralph able to crawl out and save himself.

Nevertheless, he had been badly burned, suffered smoke inhalation, and had to be rushed to the nearest hospital. As if the trauma of the fire were not enough, he was left untreated in the hospital for hours, in excruciating pain, living out his worst fears of helplessness and abandonment. To him the injustice of it felt as traumatic as the fire itself.

Two years later, Ralph was still barely able to sleep or work. His symptoms included acute and chronic stress, flashbacks, nightmares, hypervigilance, and irritability—the full post-traumatic stress disorder (PTSD) cocktail. By the time his doctor referred him to me, Ralph had given up hope of emotionally recovering.

His target image was the sight, sounds, and smell of the explosion and fireball. "I'm dead now," he uttered. The panic he felt throughout his body was off the scale.

EMDR work took him through a series of sensory memories, as he related afterward. He saw the flash of fire erupt, heard the crackling, inhaled the acrid odor, felt the intense heat and the impact of being knocked off his feet, saw himself crawl out of the window, saw the ambulance arrive, and felt the pain while he was put on a stretcher; then he saw, heard, and smelled the emergency room and the burn unit in which he had been forced to lie. He wasn't just remembering the trauma, he was *reliving* it. Images of the ER also brought up a series of memories of being left unattended as a child.

When at last the images, smells, and sounds stopped coming, I asked him to go back to the original target image to see what it elicited. Nothing came up! The sensory bombardment had vanished. His mind jumped ahead to his escape from the cellar fire, and this time he felt relief. "I'm lucky to be alive," he declared. The distressing feelings and negative cognitions were gone; but were it not for EMDR, they most likely would have haunted him for the rest of his life.

Like most of my patients, Ralph left feeling unsure about what had happened, suspicious that his reprieve would not last. We set an appointment for the following week, and when he came back, he reported that in fact he had slept soundly for the first time since the fire; that he had experienced no panic (he even went down into a neighbor's cellar to see what would happen—nothing did); and that his mood was lighter than it had been for two years.

I saw him a few times subsequently, using EMDR to help him adjust to the abrupt loss of his symptoms and go on with his life. But no further work was necessary to alleviate the residue from his trauma. It was now in his past; he was trauma free.

Ralph's first session with me had lasted an hour and a half. Throughout I felt competent, sure of myself, and confident in the marvelous technique I was privileged to have acquired. His was not the most serious traumatic experience I would encounter—far from it. In the ensuing months and years, person after person would be referred to my office, nearly destroyed by a traumatic incident, hoping that I would help them heal. A surprising number of them, it turned out, were railroad engineers.

II

MAKING THE IMPOSSIBLE POSSIBLE: HEALING TRAUMA WITH EMDR

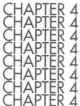

CHAPTER 4
CHAPTER 4
CHAPTER 4
CHAPTER 4
CHAPTER 4
CHAPTER 4
CHAPTER 4
CHAPTER 4 TALES FROM THE RAILS

As a kid, I was fascinated by cars and trains. By age three, I could identify the makes of most automobiles from the insignias on their hubcaps. A great thrill in my childhood was to sit in a car at a railroad crossing, or stand by the tracks, watching freight trains go by. First I'd wave to the engineer, then I'd count the cars and read the exotic names on their sides: Reading, Chesapeake & Ohio, Rock Island, Burlington—and on and on until the caboose rolled by. In my fantasies I was in the cab with the engineer, rolling toward far-off places.

It was always a special treat to travel with my family by train through Europe (and how particularly exciting it was to rise at near-forty-five-degree angles on cog railways up the Swiss and Italian Alps) and in Colorado, where at the Royal Gorge I watched the sky and vistas through the roof of the observation car as we rumbled on to places unknown.

Later, while numbed by the boredom of Hebrew school in

Forest Hills, Queens, I watched out of the window for the passing Long Island Rail Road (LIRR) trains, counting the commuter cars for diversion. The trains provided fantasies of breaking free of the restrictions and frustrations of my daily life.

Only later, as a trauma therapist, did I come to understand that the life of a railroad engineer is filled with peril. A train is a powerful weapon; it clears an indiscriminate swath through anything that lies in its path. But it doesn't choose its victims. Increasingly, desperate individuals view trains as a way to end their own lives. Ironically, many of the suicides involving engineers whom I subsequently treated took place on the same line that ran so close to my Hebrew school. As an adult and a therapist, my fantasies of becoming an engineer had long since passed over the horizon. But with EMDR, I became intimately involved with the same engineers who waved back to me in my youth, healing their occupational traumas and restoring their hopes and dreams.

ENGINEERS' TRAUMAS

When a person decides to become a railroad engineer, he—or increasingly, she—does not expect violent death to be part of the job. A cop or a fireman or someone serving on an EMT unit expects to encounter death or serious injury, and is shaken but not surprised when it happens. Train engineers understand and accept the responsibility and stress that come with the job, but they don't anticipate coming face to face with death while in their cabs.

As an engineer, your work is to drive a train, moving passengers or goods from one place or another. You're responsible for the passengers' comfort and the train's schedule—you're in command. To have someone suicidal, or inebriated, or psychotic, or fatally careless suddenly materialize in front of your hurtling engine and literally explode before your eyes is a nightmare from which you never wake up.

Imagine yourself as an executive writing a report calmly behind your desk when suddenly and without warning a man appears before you who, having eluded the building's security guards and your own secretary, crashes headfirst into your desk, killing himself instantly and splattering brains and blood across the room. It's true that the engineer might have been slightly better prepared than you were, for over 50 percent of all engineers are likely to be unwittingly involved in some accident or near miss—Bob Franke, whom you are about to meet, has done some pioneer work with the LIRR in alerting his fellow engineers to the dangers—but in all likelihood his shock would be as abiding as yours. Up until five years ago, the engineer's only recourse would have been the traditional rip-roaring night at a local bar and the well-intended advice from his colleagues, all members of a formidable fraternity, to "put it out of your head."

Today he can turn to EMDR.

EMDR HEALS AN ENGINEER

On May 21, 1995, Long Island *Newsday* ran a story about a Long Island Rail Road engineer named Bob Franke, who had noticed a pregnant woman near the tracks not far from the

Patchogue station. " 'She was walking toward me,' " the article quoted him as saying. " 'She looked sad. She looked like she had the weight of the world on her shoulders. . . . She turned toward the tracks and picked up her pace slightly. I started yelling, "Don't do it! Don't do it!" ' "

> But she did—she threw herself in front of the train. At just before 1 p.m. on March 29, the 38-year-old woman ended her life. And Bob Franke is still struggling to cope with an act the engineers fear most . . . The woman in Patchogue was the sixth person to die after being hit by a train he drove in his nearly 27 years at the controls. . . . "I can still see where the lady was standing," he said. "I can still hear the sound of her rolling under the train."

By this time I had been using EMDR with patients for two years. I had never worked with an engineer, nor with a case involving six discrete traumas, but as I read the story, I thought, *I bet I can help him.* The article spoke about post-traumatic stress disorder. I had encountered it in many of my patients; I was sure the EMDR that had worked for them would work for Bob Franke as well.

Attuned to issues of trust and appropriateness, I hesitated to approach him directly, so I called the counseling director of the LIRR's employee assistance program and asked if he would contact Bob for me. The program had existed for many years and was increasingly working with engineers involved in fatal-

ities. Some twenty people a year committed suicide by jumping in front of LIRR trains—to say nothing of accidental
deaths or injuries caused by cars stuck at intersections or children simply playing on the tracks. The director told me that he
had heard of EMDR and indeed believed it had been used
sporadically in some previous cases, but he hadn't heard about
the results. He was glad to refer Bob to me. If the engineer
agreed, I could see him.

Bob agreed.

We set our appointment for the following Sunday morning,
since I wanted to have as much time as I needed to deal with
whatever happened. Before Bob came, though, I did some
research and considerable reflecting.

Railroad trains date back to the early 1800s, and people have
been dying in front of them for just that long. An engineer sits
in front of thousands of tons of steel, often traveling in excess
of seventy miles an hour. Unlike the driver of a car, the engineer cannot swerve to prevent a collision nor apply the brakes
quickly enough to avoid impact. Instead, seeing danger, the
engineer will blow the horn and then "dump" the train, taking
his or her hand off the throttle, which automatically activates
the emergency brake. It generally takes at least a quarter of a
mile for a cruising train to stop, and by that time it's too late,
particularly if the tracks curve, the weather is inclement, or the
victim jumps suddenly onto the tracks, *wishing* to be hit. Even
though the train cannot stop abruptly, it is common for engineers to irrationally blame themselves for not reacting in time,
for not acting sooner, for having reflexes too slow or eyesight

too faulty. This is a distorted, negative cognition, but no engineer with whom I've worked is initially free of it. Unlike a car driver, who can choose a different route, an engineer must revisit the spot of the accident each day. Driving that train is the engineer's *job*.

I knew that Bob's case would be the most challenging I had yet encountered, not only because of the *number* of traumas but because the incidents spanned a long period of time.

But if I was entering uncharted territory, at least I had developed enough skills to help me navigate. All Bob had was memories, pain, and a desire to get well.

When I arrived at my office building that Sunday, Bob was already waiting, sitting in his parked car. He was a large, husky man in his late fifties, with brownish-reddish hair and a bushy mustache that reminded me of the actor Wilford Brimley, of Oat Bran commercial fame. He wore jeans and a flannel shirt over a work shirt, and even though he was obviously uncomfortable, there was a twinkle in his eye when we shook hands. His voice was gruff, and he spoke with an intensity I found compelling, even a little intimidating. I later learned that his rough exterior covered a heart that his colleagues described, with great fondness, as "mush."

We observed each other warily. Bob was suspicious of me. I suppose in his mind I was Ivy League–schooled (not true), rich (not true), and unable to relate to him or understand his feelings (not true). "I thought at first you were the kind of guy I could end up working for," Bob told me some months after the session. "I thought you didn't care." But he announced early on that, even though I was not charging him, "there is no such thing as a free cup of coffee." I quickly came to know that engineers are a unique breed, proud of their profession and their heritage, with their own language and special camaraderie—Casey Jones does not romanticize them. Bob was true to the mold.

First I asked Bob about the chronological sequence of the traumas, and then I took a thorough personal history. He was the oldest child of seven, and even as a young boy he had been his siblings' caretaker, a role he relished and had carried over to his fellow engineers—his "brothers."

"They look to me for advice," he told me—a statement of fact, not a boast. Like all novice engineers who experience a fatal incident in front of their trains, he had been inducted into the fraternity through "mediation," a ritual akin to the policemen's "choir practice," in which the subject is taken out to carouse and forget. But Bob had stopped drinking long before the first of the six accidents that had brought him to see me. I asked him about his symptoms.

He had terrible flashbacks, he told me, in which he could see every detail of each accident as clearly as when it had first happened. He was afraid to sleep for fear of nightmares, and he had frequent anxiety and panic attacks. Perhaps worst of all was his sense that at any moment another accident would occur. He was afraid of doing the job at which he was an expert and was thinking of quitting altogether to find "less dangerous" work, perhaps as a butcher, his previous profession.

All these symptoms were consistent with the symptoms of post-traumatic stress disorder (retraumatization, hypervigilance, irritability, detachment, and poor concentration are some others), about which I knew my share. I also knew that PTSD could be resolved by EMDR. But could it be cured in a man who had undergone so many traumas and been forced, by the nature of his profession, to revisit those sites on an almost daily basis?

"My wife wants to know if you're going to make me a new man," he joked, in part to test my reaction, and in part to deflect his nervousness over the unknown treatment that was to come.

"Who knows? Maybe I'll give her back the old one," I replied, "the one before the accidents, only a bit older and wiser now."

My office has a couch, three chairs, and a desk with mementos from some of my patients like paperweights and pictures. We sat across from each other in front of the desk. "What do you want to take on first? The most recent, the first, or the worst of the accidents?" I guided him.

"The most recent," he decided, and proceeded to describe it.

"There was a teenager—we later found out he was retarded—standing on the tracks. He either didn't hear the train coming or just didn't care. He had his back turned to the train. The train hit him, and he disappeared, just flew off somewhere, and all I knew was that he was hit, but I didn't know whether he was dead or where he had gone. I stopped the train—it seemed to take forever—and even though I knew the rules of the railroad said I didn't have to, I jumped out and went looking for the boy in the woods that surrounded the tracks. Who wouldn't? I wanted to see if I could do something. Anything.

"The conductor, he was with me, and pretty soon we found the boy, a good thirty feet away in the bushes, somehow still alive but bleeding and bleeding, like he had more blood in him than his body could hold. Half his ass was cut off. I knew he was alive though he wasn't screaming or anything—he must have been in shock. Anyway, I rushed back to the train to call for help and to get a blanket for him, and we covered him with it and waited till the paramedics arrived. They came fast, which probably saved his life."

He paused only momentarily. "And afterward—afterward. The cops came and did their job, which is to ask a lot of questions and make me tell the whole story from start to finish, over and over again. The bitch of it was that I had to immediately relive it all, remember it all, while I was still in a total daze, not capable of handling anything. Going home was all I wanted to do, but even that was hard." Bob told his story haltingly, but with enormous intensity and passion.

It was time to set up the protocol:

"What's the worst image that stays with you from the experience?"

"The boy standing on the tracks with his back to me," he said without hesitation.

"Any sounds or smells go with that?"

"Yeah, the thump when he hit the train."

"What is your negative belief about yourself in relation to the accident?"

He looked directly at me and said with great seriousness, "I am a terrible person. I am to blame."

All evidence to the contrary, he maintained the irrational thought that he was responsible for hitting the boy with his train. Actually, the belief "I am a murderer" had haunted him from the first fatal accident and was only reinforced with each ensuing one. The burden of self-recrimination for all those years had become terrible to bear.

We rated his SUDS level: as expected, 10. Where did he feel it in his body? "All over." Back then, for bilateral stimulation, I was using a light bar (in which lights go on and off in sequence, moving from left to right, then right to left) rather than sound, which I generally employ now. Bob stared at the lights as though wanting to melt them with his eyes.

The freshness of a trauma determines the speed by which it is played through in the patient's mind. When EMDR is used shortly after an event, the patient sees it almost frame by frame, as though he were holding a movie film up to the light. Bob's incident had happened only two months earlier, and as he processed it, the images moved sequentially in Bob's memory. Blending had begun to occur, which made the memory less intense, though still pernicious. Unless worked through, trauma can linger indefinitely, surfacing in dreams, as depression, or as panic attacks.

After Bob appeared to have processed the incident all the way through, I brought him back to the target image. The image had receded. I guided Bob to continue: "See where things go for you now when you start from the image paired with the belief, 'I am a terrible person. I am to blame.'"

Bob went back to shifting his eyes left and right, following the lights running back and forth across the bar. I let him continue for three minutes until a look of resolution appeared on his face.

"Where did you go with that?" I asked.

"My mind just ran through everything, and there was really very little left. No sounds, faint images, little emotion. My body feels relaxed. I realized that not only am I not responsible, but that I probably saved the boy's life!"

"Go with that!"

After another two minutes with the shifting light, Bob spoke again, this time with tears in his eyes. "It's over. In the past. I can go on."

"Right," I said, much moved myself. "You can go on now."

In half an hour we had conquered one trauma. There were five remaining. Since the first processing had gone so well, I encouraged Bob to go immediately to the others. We would stop only if he became exhausted or was making no progress.

We went back to the first accident, which had happened fifteen years earlier. Three teenage boys had been playing on the tracks. One had lain down across the tracks, like a character out of *The Perils of Pauline,* his head off one side, his feet off the other, only he wasn't tied to the tracks. His friends had apparently left him there, and he had fallen asleep. . . .

The train decapitated the boy and severed his legs completely. He died instantly.

Despite the fact that so many years had passed and that the boy's death was so patently accidental, the memory still packed a wallop for Bob. This made it even more surprising when the memory processed through in less than fifteen minutes. No image, no sound, no negative cognitions, no emotional or bodily distress remained!

The next event, still not "the worst," but obviously far more difficult, involved suicide. It was the case that had drawn the attention of Long Island *Newsday.*

"There was a figure on the tracks," he said. "At first I couldn't tell whether it was a man or a woman, but it kept walking *toward* the train, and pretty soon—but too late—I could tell it was a woman, a pregnant woman. God, David, she looked like my daughter! She knelt down on the track and stared up at me. I could see her eyes. I was frantically trying to stop the train, but of course I couldn't. She looked at me, made eye contact as if she wanted me to feel her suffering, and then she was under the train. I could hear the sound of it. There was no way to stop the train," he said, his voice choking. *"There was no way to stop the train!"*

Sometimes people who take pills or slit their wrists are, in effect, "experimenting" with suicide, torn between wanting death and at the same time hoping to be rescued. Ambivalence can be seen in the man threatening to jump off the ledge of a building or the woman who purposely runs her car off the road. In this case, however, it was clear that the victim had no doubts. Her actions showed full certainty; there was nothing Bob nor anyone else could have done to stop her.

I asked him what the worst image was.

"Seeing her on the tracks. Realizing she was pregnant. The eye contact."

And the negative cognition?

Similar to the others. "I am a murderer."

I am continually amazed by how trauma distorts thinking in otherwise reasonable people. The woman *wanted* to die. There was no chance Bob could have stopped that train. His culpability in the woman's death was no greater than yours or mine.

Again his emotions were horror and guilt. The distress level was back at 10—top of the scale. He felt tightness from his throat through his chest down to his stomach.

Even with the horror of this memory, it processed through in five minutes! The image lost its color, the sounds vanished, and the associated physical sensations eased and ultimately disappeared. Momentum seemed to be building as each remaining trauma was swept away. During the course of this go-round, Bob had traveled through layer upon layer of emotion. After the initial fear and guilt, he moved to anger at the woman for inflicting her suicide on him, which led to empathy and grief emerging. "I feel sad," he told me, and indeed his eyes grew watery. "That poor woman. Killing herself like that. I wish there was something I could have done to prevent it, but she didn't budge when she heard the horn. She wanted to kill herself. I did all I could."

We then came to the worst of the tragedies, an event that had taken place two years before his visit to me.

It was a snowy, icy night. A car had stalled at a railroad crossing just over a crest, which limited its visibility to Bob, and his train plowed into it broadside. The car exploded, and bits of shrapnel flew up at the train, putting Bob's own life in danger.

But he gave no thought to his safety. He heard not only the sound of the explosion but high-pitched screams. There were people in the car when it was hit. Young children!

He was able to stop the train a quarter-mile down the tracks, then raced back to the car, which was still burning. The EMTs had arrived, and Bob could see them removing bodies—no, body *parts*—from the wreckage. He made out a small arm, a foot. He could smell the burning flesh. There had been a father and two children, aged one and three, inside the car. They had all been incinerated. Bob said he observed the nightmare as though from outside his body.

"It didn't end there," Bob went on. "The family sued both me and the railroad. I had to go to two separate hearings, answer questions from three separate lawyers. In fact, I'm scheduled for another court appearance next month—two years later! Every time I testify, they treat me like a criminal. The union stuck up for me—all my buddies have been on my side. They know I couldn't prevent the crash. . . ." His voice trailed off, and he raised his head to look at me.

"It's the smell," he said. "Even today, even after all these months, I can't go to a barbecue."

When Bob finished, my first feeling was awe at his ability to carry on with his job. I had never before encountered a trauma of this magnitude (but I would treat scores more in the years to come). I was confident that EMDR would help Bob overcome its effects, but was also filled with reverence for the human spirit that can persevere in the face of such unspeakable tragedy.

This time it took Bob only fifteen minutes to process the material: the sights, the sounds, the smells, the guilt, the horror, and the distorted beliefs all vanished. Bob was imbued with a new emotional resolve.

"Those guys, all those lawyers, they're assholes," he said angrily. "I can face them in court because I did nothing wrong. If they think I did—if they so much as suggest it—they'll have to face one angry engineer!"

We spent only five minutes each on the last three accidents. In total, we had been together for no more than three hours. Bob left with a sense of exhilaration—and one last worry.

"I feel great now," he said, as we shook hands at the door. "But will it all come back? Have the memories gone forever?"

We had accomplished so much in so little time that I wasn't sure of the aftereffects. "We'll see," I said. "Time will tell. But it's quite possible your wife will have the old Bob Franke back."

Three days later he called. "The most amazing thing happened." His voice was alive with joy. "I was the engineer on my usual route, from Patchogue to Jamaica and back. But it wasn't till I was driving home after my run that it hit me. I had passed all those spots, all the places the accidents happened, and I didn't have a flashback, not one. Never even thought about them. And in the car, when I tried to remember them, I couldn't." He laughed. "And on Memorial Day, guess what my wife and I and the kids did."

I was grinning and deeply happy. "I can't imagine."

"Why," he said, "we went to a barbecue."

In the years that followed our session, I've seen Bob often. He's become one of my best friends, and our families are close. We've worked as a team to help other engineers who were the victims of traumas similar to his, well over a hundred of them. He'll contact the engineer first and explain the treatment and how it helped so many fellow engineers, then ask if it's okay for his friend David to call and explain it further. Because he is so respected, and well liked, by his peers, he is able to open the door for me to help. Unbelievable as it may seem, a few of the cases have been even more difficult than Bob's, and some have taken longer, but overall the results have been the same.

Recently I met with the president of the International Brotherhood of Locomotive Engineers, covering the United States, Canada, and Mexico, to begin a process to make EMDR accessible to engineers in need across North America. It's still often a fight to get EMDR accepted by the unions, by the U.S. Federal Railway Association (which *stresses* safety), by insurers, and by the railroad companies themselves, which can sometimes look on engineers as interchangeable parts. But we're making steady progress. And it all started with a session with Bob one Sunday in my office.

Two years ago Bob was in an automobile accident and sustained a severe head injury. His colleagues were heartbroken and rallied around him with a display of love that often brought me to tears. Bob slowly came out of it and is now 98 percent recovered, but he retired from driving trains and now spends a good deal of time being available to guide and support his fellow engineers, especially preparing newcomers for the traumas they are likely to encounter. Today this beloved man, who was so socially awkward when I first met him, gives speeches that end in standing ovations.

I try to praise him for what he does. "I don't know what to say," he tells me shyly.

"The usual response to a compliment is 'thank you,'" I reply with mock gravity.

Thanks to referrals from Bob Franke, I saw more and more engineers in my practice. All of them are memorable, yet three cases (besides Bob himself) remain the most vivid, in two instances, perhaps, because of the immense media attention lavished on them; in the third, because of the complexity of the events.

EMDR HELPS MORE ENGINEERS

BILL, STEVE, AND CHIP: CRISSCROSSING TRACKS OF TRAUMA

Bill came to see me for what I have come to consider the standard "suicide in front of the train" trauma. In this case a man in his forties sprang out from the bushes and jumped in front of the engine when it was traveling at top speed. Bill was in his mid-fifties, five foot eight, thin and muscular with salt-and-pepper hair, and despite his veteran status, this was his first such accident. The conductor of the train, a man named Tommy, happened to be with him in the engine when the train collided with the man, and the incident had bonded them to such an extent that they came in together requesting treatment. I honored this unusual request; restoring choice and control is paramount in the healing of trauma.

In one two-hour session, EMDR relieved both of them of

their traumas. Their images faded; their belief in the accident's being their fault lost its grip; the tragedy shifted from causing active trauma symptoms to being integrated as a memory.

They left immensely relieved, and a follow-up session a week later helped them reinforce their gains. A month later I received a letter from Bill thanking me in the most moving terms for my help, while on the same day, I got a call from his wife who told me that Bill was healed and that she had gotten back the man she loved. When I saw them at the annual engineers' gala dinner the following year, Bill had retired, and they had moved to Vermont, leading happy, relatively stress-free, loving lives. But before Bill retired, our paths would cross again.

Six months after I finished treating Bill, Steve came to see me with a completely different story. Steve was a Vietnam vet who had seen heavy combat during his two years in the jungle. He was a large, big-framed man with flaming red hair and a ruddy face, the kind of rough-and-tumble fellow you wouldn't want to cross if he was in a bad mood. An employee of the LIRR, though not an engineer, he told me that he had been working near the tracks when a train came hurtling by at seventy miles an hour, kicking up debris. An empty paint can had torn open his arm and shoulder, and knocked him down.

Soon after Steve's injury was reported, the railroad shut down the line in both directions until he could be moved. Steve lay between the tracks, stunned and semiconscious, waiting for medical attention. No one anticipated that when the helicopter came to medevac Steve to the hospital, the sound of the blades would trigger in him a full flashback to a thirty-year-old jungle war half a world away. Steve panicked, and it took a good hour to talk him down and carry him on a stretcher to a waiting ambulance.

I was not surprised to hear of Steve's reaction. If an area of the nervous system that has been frozen with an unprocessed trauma is reactivated by another trauma—even decades later—the victim can relive his experience as though he's actually in it. Although that sounds like a hallucination, a symptom of psychosis, it is actually a neurophysiological reaction to a triggering event. The person feels, hears, and smells the original trauma. It's terrifying—you're thrust right into a hell you thought you had escaped years ago. Often the sufferer will maintain some awareness that what he is undergoing is not really happening, but sometimes the dissociation is total, and the past trauma replaces the current reality.

I was able to guide Steve through the railroad trauma in two two-hour sessions, but we worked far longer on his Vietnam experiences and the damage it had caused in his relationship with his wife and children. For four months, we held weekly ninety-minute sessions, as Steve slowly healed from suffering he assumed he would bear the rest of his life. During breaks from therapy, we discovered that we were both longtime fans of Jackie Gleason's *The Honeymooners*. As he left my office after a particularly stressful session, Steve would give me the traditional salute of Ralph Kramden's Raccoon Lodge. "Woo-woo," he said, flipping an imaginary raccoon tail on an imaginary cap. "Woo-woo," I'd answer back.

On one occasion, Steve arrived for his session in tears. His beloved "baby" brother Chip—the weaker sibling, never married, still living with his mother, a gentle, kind soul—had been struck by a train and lay hovering near death in a Long Island hospital.

I had read the report of the accident in my morning paper, Long Island *Newsday,* but I had no idea that the injured man was Steve's brother. The shock of the news, and the possible repercussions for Steve's treatment, temporarily threw me.

Chip was an LIRR maintenance man stationed in Brooklyn, and on his way home to Long Island, he had begun to cross the tracks at the station to get to his car. He looked left, saw a train in the distance approaching the station, and walked on. But he never looked right—and stepped in front of a train bearing down on him at seventy miles per hour. Hit by a glancing blow, he was thrown thirty feet and sustained head trauma and multiple fractures. He was hospitalized in a coma. Doctors gave him less than a 50 percent chance of surviving.

Enraged, Steve stormed around my office like a runaway train. "That friggin' engineer! How the hell could he not see my brother? Why didn't he blow his whistle or dump the train?" His tears were a mixture of sorrow and rage.

He could not understand the accident was not the engineer's fault. EMDR helped considerably, but Steve couldn't fully process this new trauma, for its outcome was unresolved. There was no way to ease Steve's suspense; only time would reveal Chip's fate. We did the best we could, and he was able to calm down and pray for his brother, but we knew a lot of work remained. He agreed to keep me informed of Chip's condition and left our meeting too upset for the traditional "Woo-woo."

The next day, I got a call. I had been expecting to hear from Steve, but it was Bill. "I've got to see you," he said.

In a moment I put the pieces together. Without being told, I knew the reason for his call.

The next day a distraught Bill arrived at the office. "I hit another guy," he said, using a phrase I had noted before in other engineers. It was *he,* not "the train," who had "hit a man."

I indicated my interest and empathy. "Tell me about it."

"He was a railroad employee, one of ours, crossing the tracks. There's a curve approaching the station—my train doesn't stop there—and I blew my whistle as usual. But he didn't respond—he walked right in front of the train. One more step, and I'd have hit him full force, but it's bad enough I clipped him on his side. That horrible thump is still ringing in my ears. They don't know if he's going to live."

When treating a second trauma, there is some carryover effect from the first treatment. Although the outcome of the accident was in doubt, it only took two one-hour sessions to ease Bill's PTSD. A follow-up session a few months later revealed that all the traumatic emotions from this second accident remained resolved.

Meanwhile, I went on working with Steve. I had to resist the urge to tell him, "I know who was driving the train that hit your brother, and it wasn't the engineer's fault." Had I done so, it would have been both a violation of doctor-patient confidentiality and a clinical mistake. Steve's emotions were still too raw to allow him to put himself in the engineer's place, and he would have interpreted my work with Bill as emotional betrayal. In treating Steve I had to set aside everything I knew about Bill and his plight. And I had to empathize with Steve's anger at a man to whom I was totally sympathetic. It was an extraordinary position to be in, and I wondered if any therapist had experienced anything quite like it. I found it troubling, and hoped I wouldn't encounter another set of such coincidences soon again.

Miraculously, Steve's prayers were answered. Chip gradually recovered. With this good news, Steve was able to progressively free himself from the effects of his PTSD. After some six months, his treatment was complete. His anger had dissipated, his flashbacks had vanished, and he had forgiven the engineer. He was in control of his life, not controlled by the horrors he had witnessed and undergone. I turned my attention to other cases. Every once in a while I wondered how Steve was doing. The triple blow of his traumas (Vietnam, paint can, brother) were no small burdens for anyone to bear, EMDR notwith-standing.

Two years later, my wife, Nina, and I were entering a local Japanese restaurant when its front door opened and out strolled two men, the burly one supporting the other, who was leaning on a cane. I did not recognize either of them on the darkened street, but the heavy-set man recognized me. His hand went to the back of his head, and he flipped an imaginary raccoon tail. "Woo-woo," he shouted.

"Woo-woo," I signaled back, and Steve and I embraced.

"I want you to meet my brother," he said. I shook hands with Chip, who stood grinning at his side. "I've told him how you saved my life," Steve continued. "Maybe you can help him some time. He's still real shook up from the accident."

"Would you like to come in?" I asked Chip.

He hesitated, then plunged. "Why not?"

And so I began to treat the third man in a bizarre triangle of death and injury on the tracks. Chip had problems remembering just what had happened to him (it was hard to tell how much of his amnesia was physical, how much psychological), but at different points the emotional impact of the accident overcame him, and he would cry intensely. He had been helped enormously by the love, support, and prayers of his family, particularly Steve, and in three months of double sessions he was well on his way to healing. Some of his memory returned as well. The sound of a train whistle continued to haunt him, and he could not approach a train crossing in his car without experiencing overwhelming anxiety, fearing that a car behind him would push him onto the tracks. In time, with repeated targeting of these resistant symptoms, they vanished, too. His treatment complete, he was able to return to his mother's house in a healthier frame of mind.

Meanwhile, Steve retired and moved to Atlanta. He called one day to say that Chip was with him, and he thanked me for the help I had given both of them. When he hung up, I felt exhilarated, almost giddy. My hand instinctively reached to the back of my head, and I flicked my fingers upward.

Woo-woo, I thought, and opened the door to my next patient.

ERIC: THE FAMILY IN THE HEADLIGHT

By 1998, treating railroad engineers had become a specialty of mine. Not only did they come to me (often introduced by Bob

Franke), but sometimes I would seek them out. I never approached them directly, but I used contacts within the engineer fraternity to let them know I was available. Thus when I read the terrible news story that a train had hit and killed a woman and her three young children, I knew that the engineer, a man named Eric, would be devastated, so I used my contacts to try to reach him. (Engineers keep tabs on the "worst incidents," and Eric was high on the list.) Eric's brother inadvertently added to my resolve when he said on a radio show, "He'll never be the same. The image will be with him forever." His statement strengthened my resolve to find Eric. Given the opportunity, I knew I could help him let it go.

Word came back to me that Eric was receiving help and that he was doing okay. But three months later, the chairman of his union local called. Could I see Eric? *Could* I? I left my morning open, not knowing how much time would be needed, and the union chairman accompanied him in—then sat patiently in my waiting room until the session was finished.

Eric told me the details quite calmly, though he was obviously under great internal strain. The accident had happened at night, and the eerie image—the train's light suddenly picking out the woman and children standing with their backs to him on the tracks—haunted him. He wondered whether it was suicide or an accident, as the papers reported. He thought he had gotten over the worst of it by himself, but one night he had a nightmare where he saw four ghostly heads coming at him with a moaning sound. The next day when he climbed into the cab and sat at the controls, he began to shake uncontrollably.

Panic followed, so severe that he had to be helped from the train. This incident was frightening enough for him to request more help.

When we started EMDR, Eric was stuck with one frozen image: the woman and children in the faint headlight. But then the image was replaced by another, then another. The woman and the children. The bodies exploding. The sight and smell of blood. The sound of the screams and the grinding of brakes, followed by a ghastly silence.

Eric had memories of the aftermath, too, when the police interrogated him. It was their job, he knew, but he felt like a mugging victim being accused of assault.

Our EMDR session lasted two and a half hours. As he approached resolution, Eric saw the faint images of the four victims rise peacefully into heaven. He heard ethereal voices saying, "We're with God now." Then it was over; his SUDS scale was 0, and his mind, body, and spirit were calmed. As amazing as this seems, when he came in a week later for a follow-up, we could find no lingering trauma, though I probed hard for signs. He had passed the scene of the accident, offered a prayer and suffered no flashbacks, and gone on with his life.

MAX: CARNAGE IN LONG ISLAND

On December 7, 1993, train number 1256, the 5:33 P.M. out of Pennsylvania Station, departed for its evening suburban run. Between the New Hyde Park and Merillon stations, a man named Colin Ferguson, sitting three cars from the front, arose, took out an automatic weapon, and began to fire randomly at passengers, working his way systematically toward the front car. If not for the bravery of the passengers who eventually wrestled him to the ground, many more would have been injured or killed. Carolyn McCarthy, whose husband was killed and son wounded on the train, was later elected to Congress after campaigning on the issue of gun control. Greater security measures were instituted by the railway. Years later, the memory still haunts Long Island Rail Road commuters. Some twenty passengers and the conductor were later treated by colleagues of mine using EMDR.

The engineer of 1256 was a mild-mannered, pleasant thirty-eight-year-old bodybuilder with massive shoulders and neck named Max, who happened to be a good friend of Bob Franke's. From his perch in the engine car, he did not see the killings, but he could hear the sounds of mayhem behind him. He figured that a robbery was going on, and that the best thing to do was to immediately call the police, then stop at the next station—Merillon—and wait for them to arrive.

But there was a problem. The Merillon station can accommodate only eight cars, not the ten making up train 1256. Max knew that if he opened the doors, people in the last two cars, trying to exit, might fall down a steep embankment and be injured or killed. On the other hand, keeping the doors closed would trap the passengers inside the train until help arrived. Faced with this conundrum, he opted to keep the doors closed.

By the time the police and paramedics arrived at the scene, the massacre was over. Max climbed out of the engine car and moved down the platform, seeing for the first time what had really happened. Police and paramedics were swarming through the cars, but he was struck by the particularly horrible sight of an Asian girl blown to pieces, an image that would stalk him in the coming years. He broke into a cold sweat, his knees buckled, and he had to cling to a post to keep from collapsing onto the platform.

Ferguson was eventually tried and convicted of murder, and the incident became a grim moment in history for the railroad and the community. Max went on with his job; he thought he had gotten over the shock. Then, six years later to the day, as he approached the 5:33 train that he had driven for all those years, he caught a glimpse of the number on the engine: 1256. It was the first time he had drawn that engine since the incident, and the sight of it threw him into such severe panic that he could not board the train. Everything came back to him, including the image of the Asian girl, and he was suddenly overcome with guilt. *It was my fault that those people died. I made the wrong decision. If I had opened the doors, none of this would have happened.*

This was the negative cognition he carried when, on Bob Franke's urging, he came to see me. As we worked together, he consciously faced for the first time the fact that he himself could have been killed; he had previously blocked it out. And in a single two-hour session of EMDR, the trauma was 95 percent resolved! (The remaining issues were resolved in another session a week later.) The image of the car became blurred and then disappeared; the sounds of the screams were muted. Yes, he is still saddened by the tragedy; the memory has not been erased. Max had long had a claustrophobic reaction to crowds, and during the processing he connected that reaction, for the first time, with the incident. His claustrophobia is now gone as well.

EMDR therapists have the privilege to travel with their clients from the moment of their horror to the moment of their healing, a journey complete with spiritual imagery, emotions, and bodily experience. In this way, I "rode the cab" with Max, Eric, Chip, Steve, Bill, Bob, and many others. Their dramas and fears were almost palpable. Like my EMDR colleagues around the world, I'm exhilarated by knowing that I'll be able to help my clients let go of their suffering. From discussions with other EMDR practitioners, I've discovered that we all share the quiet pleasure of knowing that at the outset our patients can't possibly imagine how EMDR will change their lives at warp speed, and how at the end we'll be able to tell them, "I believed this would happen all along." These are the secret thoughts of therapists that bring us joy. For in treating our patients we're regularly honored to enter the strange world ruled by the miracles of the mind.

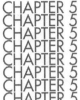

CHAPTER 5
CHAPTER 5
CHAPTER 5
CHAPTER 5
CHAPTER 5
CHAPTER 5
CHAPTER 5
CHAPTER 5 THE MIND IS A MAGICIAN:
THE PROCESS OF DISSOCIATION

Why does EMDR work so well in the treatment of trauma? Identifying the target using the protocol (target image, cognitions, emotion, and body experience) identifies the location where the trauma is stuck in the nervous system. Applying bilateral stimulation reactivates the system, removes the blocks, and allows for reconnection and healing.

The mind can act like a magician—it can make painful memories "vanish." By the process known as *dissociation,* the conscious mind cloaks intolerable emotions and memories, sometimes through forgetfulness, sometimes through a wall of amnesia, sometimes even by splitting into more than one personality. Dissociation does not eliminate the effects of a trauma; it merely buries them. We may not consciously feel their effects, may often not even remember the original trauma itself. But although hidden by this defense, they remain active, affecting the way we think, the way we feel both emotionally and physically, the way we speak, our relationships, the way we behave, the way we *are.*

Trauma and dissociation go together like hand and glove—and EMDR can help to ease off the glove. Only by getting to the heart of the trauma, becoming aware of it, and seeing it clearly can we overcome its force—only then can we change. Changes this dramatic need to take place carefully and sensitively. Old defenses have to be carefully eliminated so that more adaptive ones can take their place.

DYSFUNCTIONAL DISSOCIATION

When a person is faced with real or perceived danger, the body reacts: the flow of adrenaline increases, respiration speeds up or momentarily stops, the skin flushes or pales, and the mind is shocked, first registering and then often forgetting the traumatic event. Severe trauma is simply too much to integrate. We reflexively protect ourselves from it—we blot it from our consciousness. Therapists used to call this phenomenon *repression*. Now it's more commonly referred to as dissociation.

Not all dissociation is dysfunctional. Indeed, if we were in touch with what we were feeling at all times, we'd be bombarded and unable to function. When your mind wanders in a lecture and you realize you don't have any idea what you've just heard, that's dissociation. When you turn the pages of a book and have no recollection of what was on the prior page, that's dissociation. When you find yourself driving on a highway and suddenly realize you haven't been *conscious* of driving for some time, that's a form of dissociation. But pathological dissociation is a reaction to trauma.

How we react to trauma, and *where* we react in our bodies, depends on the level of development of our nervous system and the severity of the trauma. An infant's system is immature and vulnerable. An infant who is repeatedly abused by a parent will dissociate the trauma, yet it will mold her entire life, and its aftershocks will likely break through by adolescence or adulthood. A child of five or ten who is similarly abused will be deeply affected, but her greater level of development may alter the nature of the damage.

Similarly, if you as an adult lose a loved one, you may well, for a brief time, feel that the departed is still alive, speak of him in the present tense, and even "see" him walking down the street. This is a "normal" dissociative process. Your cognitive brain takes in the information that the person is dead, but your emotional brain still struggles to grasp it. Only gradually will the awareness of your loved one's death filter from your "thinking" brain into your whole nervous system, allowing you to make the transition to the next stages—grief, anger, depression, acceptance, healing. But if you suffer a severe trauma—in combat, for instance, or such as Bob or Steve or Bill underwent—you may not be able to process the trauma without outside help. It is then that EMDR becomes invaluable.

THE UBIQUITY OF ABUSE

Whole societies may experience denial, particularly regarding the abuse of children. Its effects are so devastating, and what it says about us as human beings so threatening, that we prefer to view the beating or the sexual exploitation of children as isolated events, manifestations of depravity that no "normal" community could countenance. As Dr. Judith Lewis Herman writes in her landmark book, *Trauma and Recovery* (1992, pp. 7, 8),

> The study of psychological trauma has repeatedly led into realms of the unthinkable and foundered on fundamental questions of belief. . . . To study psychological trauma is to come face to face with both human vulnerability in the natural world and with the capacity for evil in human nature. To study psychological trauma means bearing witness to horrible events. When the events are natural disasters or "acts of God," those who bear witness sympathize readily with the victim. But when the traumatic events are of human design, those who bear witness are caught in the conflict between victim and perpetrator. It is morally impossible to remain neutral in this conflict. The bystander is forced to take sides.
>
> It is very tempting to take the side of the perpetrator. All the perpetrator asks is that the bystander do nothing. He appeals to the universal desire to see, hear, and speak no evil. The victim, on the contrary, asks the bystander to share the burden of pain. . . .
>
> In order to escape accountability for his crimes, the perpetrator does everything in his power to promote forgetting. Secrecy and silence are the perpe-

trator's first line of defense. If secrecy fails, the perpetrator attacks the credibility of his victim. If he
cannot silence her absolutely, he tries to make sure
that no one listens. . . . After every atrocity one can
expect to hear the same predictable apologies: it
never happened; the victim lies; the victim exagger-
ates; the victim brought it upon herself; and in any
case it is time to forget the past and move on. The
more powerful the perpetrator, the greater is his
prerogative to name and define reality, and the more
completely his arguments prevail.

Adults exercise enormous power over young children, and
no perpetrator is more guaranteed to impose silence on his
victim than an adult who abuses a child. For the youngest of
children can't speak out, can't react (because her—or his—
brain is still insufficiently formed to understand, let alone interpret, what has happened), can do nothing to escape from her
persecutor and from the trauma itself. She can do only one
thing: dissociate from it. A child—age six or seven, say—often
will "float out of her body" when she is being abused, observing but not feeling anything, and trying to disappear (a symptom described by abuse victims at every age). Often, in fact, she
gets her wish, and her core person is lost deep inside, sometimes permanently.

Whether we deny it or not, child abuse is prevalent in our
society, just as it was throughout the millennia that preceded
ours. There are usually no witnesses save the perpetrator and

the victim. We can only guess at the numbers of cases, knowing that the existing reports are reduced in numbers by fear, guilt, shame, and the forgetting through dissociation. Sigmund Freud wrote in 1896 in *The Aetiology of Hysteria* that, "at the bottom of every case of hysteria there are *one or more occurrences of premature sexual experience,* [italics added] occurrences which belong in the earliest years of childhood." Yet he later recanted (perhaps threatened into his own denial, perhaps pressured by a society that asserted that such things did not happen) and described such occurrences as fantasies caused by "hysteria," a condition of the times that parallels symptomatically what we now call traumatic stress syndrome. Although memory is inexact and sometimes fallible, my experience has been that dissociation is not present without a very good reason—the person *needs* to forget. Controversy rages about "false memory syndrome," since some unscrupulous therapists have directed suggestible patients to trauma without sufficient basis. But this label has also been used to deny recovered abuse memories, even when they are verified.

It is a truism that human beings are capable of exquisite kindness as well as rank depravity. We carry in us the potential for the best and the worst. Somewhere in every Mother Teresa there is a dark side, in every criminal the capacity for redemption. All of us struggle to restrain our aggressive impulses and cultivate our humanistic ones; not all of us succeed. And our capacity to do harm can be most tragic when it is directed at our own daughters and sons. As a therapist, I see these two forces at war with each other in the patients I treat, as well as in myself. It's no surprise to me when "the boy next door" deto-nates a massive explosive in front of a populated government building, or when a murderer devotes his prison life to helping fellow inmates.

CONNIE: TRIGGERED BY THE LIGHT

I have observed that EMDR practitioners tend to discover more dissociation in their patients than other psychotherapists. Depression, anxiety, and behavioral problems, which many therapists treat symptomatically, are often *dissociative identity disorders*—trauma-based neurophysiological ways of escaping something too overwhelming to confront. For therapists and patients alike, it is important to remember that such extreme splitting is not true madness—quite the contrary, it is in fact a form of sanity, a last-ditch means of avoiding the traumatic abyss. Suddenly touching on a traumatic memory can cause immense disorientation. Inexpertly applied, EMDR can accelerate this process.

Before I was trained in EMDR, I had worked with Connie for three productive years on her symptoms of panic and depression. I knew I had not reached the core of her problems and sensed that something profoundly troubling had occurred when she was young. During treatment she recalled that her father, a police officer, had sometimes struck her when she was a little girl, and she needed help to be shown that her overwhelming fears and self-criticism were conncted to those incidents.

I noticed that Connie would always cringe when I turned on a lamp or opened the window blinds. (She was fine if the room remained consistently lighted.) She was a slim, well-dressed woman in her late fifties, with short dark brown hair who seemed to protect herself by hunching over and averting her eyes, no matter how innocuous the conversation. I was struck primarily with how *clean* she was, how well manicured and coiffed, like a little girl trying to please her parents.

Looking for a breakthrough when I returned from facilitator training, I decided to see how Connie responded to EMDR and asked her to choose an issue on which we would work.

"My sensitivity to light," she said.

Light sensitivity is not a common target, but she chose a recent experience where light bothered her. For her negative cognition, she located "Danger!" Her SUDS level was 8, and she felt fear in her chest and extremities. With eyes moving left to right and back again, she quickly reverted to an early memory.

"I have a memory from when I was five," she told me. "I'm in the street with my father, looking up at a hospital window. My mother's behind that window, and I'm not allowed to visit her. The sunlight is glinting off the glass so I can't even see her."

Her voice became low and tight. "Now we're back home, my father and me, and I'm in the bathtub and he's washing me, all over, with a washcloth. It's warm in the tub, cozy." She shook her head, bewildered. "Something bad is happening, I feel a sensation between my legs. My father," she said, and her voice rose in terror, "my father is putting his finger inside me!"

She became extremely agitated. "It didn't happen!" she

screamed. "It couldn't have happened. Why did I say that? Why am I *thinking* it?" She stood and began to pace, as disjointed images—of her father and her in the apartment, again in the tub only this time she's six, in the kitchen—spilled out of her memory in an avalanche. I had never seen such distress, so I tried to bring her back into the present moment.

"Connie, where are you going to be later in the day?"

"I love him!" she cried. "He didn't do those awful things. He couldn't. He loved me."

"Connie, we'll deal with this together, step by step. Try to give it time."

She returned to the chair, and her breathing slowed, and soon she was able to talk to me rationally, although she was still visibly shaken. We went back to familiar issues to ground her— her complaints about her job, her conflicts with her husband— and she left my office calmly, if unsteadily, promising to call if she became overwhelmed. We arranged for a phone contact the next day and a second session later on in the week.

She returned to my office in a somber state, after a particularly tumultuous three days, her sleep disrupted by nightmares. This was unusual for her; generally she felt relieved after our sessions and slept well. I did not use EMDR with her for that session or for several subsequent weeks as we worked on grounding and discussing what had emerged, but eventually she wanted to try it again. Patently it activated something that we could not reach through conventional talk therapy.

Connie steeled herself as we began our session, and returned to her image.

"The light."

"What's the distress level?"

"Ten."

"Observe where your mind goes," I advised, slowly tracking my hand back and forth.

"It's—coming from my left—from my parents' bedroom door. I'm lying in my bed, and I see the light streaming into my room." Once more she shook her head in denial. "I know this didn't happen—*it didn't happen!*—my father's standing at my door. He's walking over to my bed. Now he's lying on top of me. He's sticking his penis in me. And it hurts. It hurts!"

She became increasingly dissociated from her surroundings as her memories grew more real. "I'm in the room there with him. I'm there *now*. I can hardly breathe. He's so heavy. I can't move. I can't cry, but I want to cry. I'm leaving my body. Watching from outside myself—from the wall."

She curled up in the chair, cowering, and then she began to wail, a terrible rasping sound filled with terror and rage. Vietnam veterans, I knew, experienced similar flashbacks, crawling on the floor to get away from the horrors they were reliving. Connie was reliving a memory so powerful and so terrifying that it transformed her into a helpless five-year-old, unable to escape from the monster who was attacking her.

"Keep away from me!" she screamed. "You stay right there!"

I kept my cool and spoke soothingly.

"Where are we now?"

She gasped out the words. "In my house."

"Who am I?"

"You're my father!" Her eyes flashed such malice and terror that I braced myself.

It would have been a mistake to challenge her then. It would only increase her agitation, and what I wanted to do was bring her safely back to her present-day adult self.

My next question came on a hunch. "Who's the president?" It brought her up short. "Roosevelt."

"Roosevelt?" I said slowly. "Are you sure?"

I could see her begin to come back. Her hands relaxed, and her posture softened. Her mouth formed a single word.

"Clinton."

"Yes," I said softly. "Bill Clinton is president now." I walked over to my desk and picked up the newspaper. "See, it's 1995."

She stood silently, trembling and bewildered.

"And who am I?" I asked.

"David."

"Yes. David."

She sat down across from me. "Where was I?" she said cautiously.

Experience later taught me that when a patient denies such painful events, probably something actually did occur. If Connie had accepted without protest the fact of her father's incest, her memories might have been less convincing. Months later, she asked questions of her mother and sister that she could not previously have asked—would not have *known* to ask—and received corroboration of her father's actions.

But that knowledge only opened the door. Eight more months of intensive EMDR processing followed, at times activating intense agitation for her. Two other alter states emerged, one aggressive and the other robotic, devoid of feelings. She was suffering from dissociative identity disorder (DID). More and more memories surfaced of terrifying, humiliating abuses. (When her mother was in the hospital, for instance, her father insisted that she become "the woman of the house" even though she was only five, and he beat her when dinner was not prepared or if his clothes had not been properly put away.)

Eventually, the images began to fade, and Connie reintegrated the selves, one by one, each with a tearful farewell. She was able to discuss with me the crimes her father had perpetrated. Still, she was not fully healed when circumstances forced her to move to California and our therapy sessions ended.

I looked on Connie's departure with mixed feelings. So much had changed for her, beyond my expectations, yet her recovery had not been completed. Initially I had been in over my head, and I knew it. For me, it had been at times frightening, at times humbling, but always an incredible education. I had learned that with EMDR, dissociative conditions caused by sexual abuse in childhood could be healed in a time period previously inconceivable, though hardly at the "warp speed" I would see later in discrete trauma cases.

TRAUMA AND THE NERVOUS SYSTEM

The human nervous system develops incrementally, which means that children are less protected against trauma than adults. An infant responds to stimuli with his or her *reptilian* brain, or hindbrain, the primitive part of the brain that regulates breathing, blood flow, and all the other basic life functions. The *limbic* or mid- or mammalian brain is also active from the start, generating the beginnings of the fight-or-flight response, later developing as the seat of the emotional self. Gradually, the *thinking* brain, the neocortex or forebrain, comes online, enabling us to think, to reason, and to understand abstract ideas and observe ourselves. PTSD has not been observed in mammals other than primates; less-developed creatures seem to have been spared the glitches that can occur with a highly developed brain—a thinking brain.

So an infant registers trauma in the primitive brain. A slightly older baby will react in the gradually more developed brain; a child begins to have access to the thinking brain, though he will not react as an adult does—sophisticated comprehension is well beyond his means. When the information-processing connections are broken or don't develop, which often happens in cases of intense or repeated trauma, then dissociation frequently results. If the trauma occurs in adulthood, the sufferer will "know" that the incident and its danger are over yet will nevertheless feel an overriding dread. But a child "forgets" what has happened to her, and it is only later, in adolescence and adulthood, that bits and pieces of the traumatic experience may emerge.

A classic example of childhood trauma abuse reemerging can be seen when a woman in her twenties, thirties, or forties suddenly begins to experience strange, unexplainable symptoms: tingling or pressure occurring in her erogenous zones;

frightening images flashing from nowhere; panic inexplicably surfacing. In severe cases, she will discover that she has dissociative identity disorder (DID) and alter states of different ages and personalities. These selves can be male or female, children and adults, all within the same individual, who "come out" depending on the situation. (In a case I know of, one of the personalities, a man, was a heavy drinker; another, a woman, was allergic to alcohol.) People who suffer from this condition will often find clothes in their closets that they don't remember buying, or notes that they don't recall writing, with unrecognizable handwriting. This loss of reality is dissociation, but again it is not psychosis. It is the desperate self-protective maneuver of a person who has been cruelly abused, fighting to maintain her equilibrium. A psychotic is out of touch with reality, but each of the personalities in a DID sufferer is in touch in the context of his or her world.

EGO STATES

A more common—and less dramatic—form of dissociation is the phenomenon of *ego states,* also called *separate selves.* To some degree or another, we all have distinct aspects of ourselves that can sometimes seem to not really be "us" but rather are parts of us that we experience in the third person. In a simple example, we can be both the critic and the criticized simultaneously. "You stupid idiot!" we'll say aloud to ourselves when we mess up, or "How could you have made such a mistake?"

   Each of us can be both adult and child, jury and criminal,

doctor and patient, teacher and student—and yes, therapist and client. In the course of our daily lives, we unconsciously assume roles befitting our situation, adopting a demeanor, a tone of voice, a look, and an aspect that best suits the circumstance. A fireman is only a fireman when he is putting out fires; he usually takes off his slicker and his "inner uniform"—his protective layer—when he returns home. Ego states include our child self, adolescent self, competent adult self, critical self, and criticized self, among countless others.

STAN: HEALING THE CRITICAL SELF

By accessing ego states, a therapist can help patients locate and work with sides of themselves that are lost or out of reach. The mind's eye is adept at working with these selves, and when it is enhanced with EMDR, amazing things can happen.

Recently I treated Stan, an executive who, although happily married and professionally successful, was unable to shake his low self-esteem and passivity. His mother had always compared him harshly to his father and brother, and he was stuck with the belief that he was worthless and always would be. Activating him with bilateral sound stimulation, I suggested that his negative, critical self might be outside the door, in the waiting room. I guided him to call in this self and tell me when he appeared. Almost immediately he reported that he could see this hostile self. My first question was an effort to establish where in the developmental scale this self fell.

"How old is he?"

"Six."

"What's he wearing?"

"Shorts and a T-shirt."

"What's his facial expression?"

"His face is fierce. He's mad at me."

I guided Stan to ask this self if he would talk directly with me. Giving him this option granted him choice and control, both of which are essential elements in trauma healing.

I asked the aggressive self whether he was genuinely strong or really felt wounded and vulnerable.

"I'm suffering."

"Would you like to try some EMDR?" I asked.

"Sure. Why not? What do I have to lose?"

"Can you hear the bilateral sound that your overall self is hearing now?"

"Yes."

"I want you to process what is bothering you and let me know what happens," I guided.

This young, critical self began his own processing, and within a few minutes he was able to be more benign.

"Can you now use your determination and energy for constructive purposes, helping yourself and your overall self?"

"Yes."

I now spoke to Stan's adult self. "Can you look at this child self and see if you can feel compassion toward him?"

"I see myself putting my arm around my six-year-old self, who has dropped his attack and now appears vulnerable," Stan said. "My formerly critical self has merged back into me. I feel more integrated, more at peace, more confident."

I encouraged Stan to go with these feelings and let the bilateral stimulation strengthen them. When we returned to the target image, it had shifted dramatically, and the SUDS level, which had been stuck at 7, dropped to a 2. This approach may sound unreal or hokey, but I invite you to try it for yourself. Just imagine that your critical self is in the next room, call him or her in, observe the age and dress, and let the dialogue begin.

OTHER REACTIONS TO TRAUMA

Generalized anxiety attacks or panic attacks are usually not thought of as trauma-based conditions. Yet panic can be a dissociated emotional memory of something that the person experienced during an earlier overwhelming situation. A girl who slept in her parents' room until the age of five, immobilized by terror and shame by the sights, sounds, and smells of the sex act (known as the primal scene), may as an adult suddenly experience panic in an elevator, a bathroom, or an airplane. Untreated, her panic may spread into fear of going out of the house, known as agoraphobia. Genetics plays a significant role in the formation of personality, as well as in vulnerability to anxiety, depression, obsession, and addiction. But when EMDR targets the symptoms, a trauma history frequently emerges.

We've seen that symptoms can emerge soon after a trauma or lie dormant for months or even years. They may seem unrelated to the source trauma, manifesting as physical pain or numbness, diminished pleasure from sex or recreation, psychomotor retardation, feelings of worthlessness, confusion, or intrusive thoughts of death. PTSD has many guises—and many degrees of severity. One's reactions may be normal (memories, mild anxiety, nondebilitating fear), pathological (dissociation), or extremely pathological (DID), though these boundaries are often hazy. It's impossible to get through life without experiencing depression, and if the depression lifts within a few days or a week, it is normal and appropriate, even if the cause goes unrecognized. But severe symptoms that last for months or recur regularly indicate clinical depression that can be painful, debilitating, and potentially dangerous. We tend to believe that our joy and sadness are determined externally more than internally, yet hopelessness and helplessness are often present even when life circumstances are favorable.

Humans are extraordinarily adaptive. Given enough time and support, we can overcome many traumas and their attendant symptoms by ourselves. Indeed, we intuitively recognize that our reactions are transient—in itself a sign of good health. *I'll bounce back,* we think, or, *That knocked me down, but I'll get back on my feet.* Still, despite our varied levels of hardiness, the severity of one trauma or a series can exceed our ability to adapt and recover. This is where therapy comes in.

EMDR AND THE TREATMENT OF TRAUMA

Talk therapy—whether it be psychoanalysis, family systems therapy, cognitive therapy, behavior modification, or some other form—enters the system through the cortical region of the brain, the seat of logic and thought. But trauma deeply affects the mammalian or emotional brain (which is difficult to access through talking), the reptilian brain, and the body (which is inaccessible to verbal interchange).

EMDR appears not only to have access to these regions, but to have the ability to change them. When patients describe *and feel* an image or a negative memory, they're activating the place where it is held in the nervous system—in the body, hindbrain, midbrain, and forebrain. Words can't describe something that happened when we were incapable of speech, but by activating images, sounds, smells, and body sensations, we gain access to the primitive brain. Evoking the emotions associated with a sensory experience can activate the primitive responses allied with trauma. What emerges is not only in the brain but also in the body (in my work, I don't isolate the brain from the body), for the brain is really just the central switching station of the nervous system. Thus EMDR is a "bottom up" therapy: it activates body memory, which travels through the primitive regions of the brain and ultimately arrives at the thinking brain for final analysis and resolution. By contrast, talk therapy is a "top down" approach: information enters through the cortical brain with limited access to the emotional brain and even less access to the hindbrain and the body. Is it any wonder that talk therapy alone accomplish such limited success with body-centered conditions like PTSD?

The EMDR protocol activates unprocessed information in the nervous system. Left-right stimulation can free up this material, whether it has been stuck there for two weeks or twenty years. Dr. Strickgold's study of rapid eye movement

(REM) sleep—necessary sleep cycles that a sleeper goes through numerous times a night—shows that certain events and feelings, stimulated both externally and internally, are processed nightly deep inside the brain.

Experiences that arise in EMDR often have a kind of dreamlike quality. The therapist uses verbal communication to set up the protocol, to regulate the flow of images and feelings, and at times even to direct it. The patient uses talk to describe what is happening: the memories, the emotions, the body experiences. But the essential healing work goes on internally, quickly and powerfully, often without words, in a way that even the patient is not fully aware of, let alone understands.

Occasionally only a few words beyond the setup are needed. I recently treated a deeply troubled sixteen-year-old who was unable or unwilling to talk about what was hurting him. Still, he agreed to undergo EMDR, with the stipulation that he wouldn't have to discuss anything unless he chose to.

"I want you to think about what's bothering you now," I told him.

A mumble. "Yeah."

"Can you see it?"

"Yes."

"Is it bringing up feelings inside you?"

"Yes. But I don't want to tell you—"

"You don't have to. In fact, it's better if you don't. Just rate your distress level. What would it be if ten is the worst and zero is no problem?"

"A ten."

"Where do you feel it in your body?"

"All over."

Silence.

He put on the headphones, listened to bilateral rock music, and processed for fifteen minutes without uttering a word. Afterward, when we checked his target image the first time, his distress was down to a 4. The second check yielded a 1 and the third produced 0 distress. Could such results be accomplished with any other modality of therapy? No way. I realized that something was going on deep inside my patient, something profound. I'll never know what it was. Did I have to? Not if I knew that his healing changed his everyday life. And his mother reported his mood and behavior improved dramatically after our session.

THE ROLE OF THE THERAPIST

This is not to say that EMDR works in a vacuum. EMDR seems straightforward, but in practice it is very technical. The therapist must direct the protocol and guide the patient, and once the system starts working, unexpected complications often emerge. True resolution is also complex, both mentally and systemically. The therapist has to know what he's doing diagnostically and recognize the forces that come into play throughout the process. And despite the internal nature of EMDR, the therapist must have acute listening skills to take in the multilevel communications that go on during the treatment.

Take ego-state work. In one session, Terry, a thirty-seven-year-old manicurist, was processing through an ego state, her critical self ("you're a failure"), while another self—a hidden "spiritual" part of herself in opposition to it—seemed to come out of nowhere, and a struggle ensued. At another time, a shaming self lurked behind her critical self, and it was hard to delineate and negotiate between the two. In time, the two selves found common ground and reintegrated. An EMDR therapist needs to know how to locate and access these disparate selves and how to interact with them. For this process, diagnostic and treatment skills are crucial.

Alan, for example, had a frightened child-self that was intimidated by his aggressive adolescent ego state. They needed separate healing before they could be brought together for a supervised give-and-take negotiation over issues of assertiveness and sensitivity. Eventually the process helped bring Alan inner harmony, and he was able to resolve his internal struggles.

The accelerated integration potential of EMDR offers opportunities for achieving a more profound level of conflict resolution than can be realized with most talk psychotherapies. EMDR activates the parts of the nervous system where the blocking trauma is held and then fosters its release and resolution.

But the process of integration is delicate. (In some DID patients, it may be better not to try to attempt it.) The more damaged the patient, the more support the therapist must lend. Even a badly scarred person with virtually no self-esteem will have some areas of strength. The question "Do you have an image of yourself as a competent adult?" will solicit that picture (often to the patient's great surprise), and the patient can more deeply grasp this image and feeling by strengthening it with the aid of bilateral stimulation.

The biggest issue for deeply traumatized patients is always trust. And in a person who was abused by someone upon whom she once relied for nurturance, initial distrust of the therapist is appropriate. A patient will correctly say early in treatment, "Why should I trust you—or anybody?" It is the normal response for those who have experienced the abnormality of abuse. When a patient undergoes a traumatic event as an adult, trust is somewhat easier to establish—but the treatment has complexities and problems of its own, since it often uncovers traumas from earlier in life.

CHAPTER 6
CHAPTER 6
CHAPTER 6
CHAPTER 6
CHAPTER 6
CHAPTER 6
CHAPTER 6
CHAPTER 6 ALMOST TOO GOOD TO BE TRUE:
HEALING ADULT TRAUMA

Most traumatic events in adult life are discrete, once-in-a-lifetime events that can last a mere second or a number of hours. An automobile crash or a mugging are two examples; the sudden death of a parent due to heart attack or accident is another. The severity of the trauma, and therefore the relative ease of treatment, is different in each instance. Another variable is the makeup of the traumatized person, both genetic and psychological. Some people seem to get through horrendous events with few if any symptoms; others are traumatized by incidents that, to most others, might be tolerable. To some degree, all of us sustain traumas in our lifetimes. (Even rejection by a boyfriend or girlfriend leaves its mark.) All of us will react differently, though we share a range of common symptoms.

War is among the foremost causes of trauma in adults, for civilians as well as soldiers. Wartime traumas may be discrete (the soldier wounded on his first day of action) or extended and repeated (the Vietnam "grunt" fighting in the jungle for years on end). Neurologists have demonstrated through brain scans that in people subjected to protracted trauma the hippocampus—that region of the brain that takes in objective facts and relays them to the amygdala for emotional response and the neocortex for "analysis"—shrinks, reducing and impeding many levels of brain function. In adult Holocaust survivors, victims of arguably the worst trauma inflicted by man on man, the capacity to heal psychologically, neurologically, and symptomatically is dramatically different even from that of Vietnam veterans because the nature of the trauma was so profound and unique.

EMDR can heal such profound traumas, if not completely, at least to some degree, though in these cases the term *warp speed* is relative. Compared with talk therapy, the healing process will go far more quickly; I have seen a two-year treatment of once- or twice-weekly sessions with EMDR accomplish what twenty years of most therapies cannot. The more protracted the trauma, the more difficult it is to resolve. Still, EMDR, miraculous as it is, is not a panacea. Sometimes psychic wounds are simply too deep to fully cure.

DISCRETE TRAUMA: THE DEATH OF A LOVED ONE

When an eighty-year-old parent dies of natural causes, his or her adult children will mourn, but it is unlikely they will be traumatized. The daughter or son *expects* the death—it is in the natural order of things—and the child will go through the stages of mourning and grief, emerging resolved on the other side. But if the mourning extends too long, if the person cannot let go and recover, then a pathological symptom has emerged, one that is likely driven by earlier trauma and is in need of treatment.

When a death is sudden, these dynamics change. Now the unexpected plays a prominent role, and will invariably result in acute trauma. (Unexpectedness is a crucial factor in PTSD.) The eleven-year-old whose father dies of a heart attack will be affected differently from the fifty-one-year-old whose father also suddenly passes away. The adult survivor will still have to go through the multistage healing process—it's just that the loss is less shocking, less traumatic. But if the parent is ill for a long time, even though death is expected, the accumulated effect of the illness often increases the dimension of the trauma.

Again, each individual will respond differently to a loved one's passing, depending on his or her constitution (genetic makeup and brain chemistry) and life experience. Still, the reaction will typically fall within a certain range, and if it doesn't, the therapist's antennae will sense it. If for example, that eleven-year-old whose father suddenly died of a heart attack exhibits no symptoms and doesn't seem traumatized, the therapist will be alerted to look deeper. Every action leads to a reaction. If it doesn't happen directly, it will come out sideways. It can emerge somatically, in headaches or backaches, or behaviorally, in workaholism or numbing out. The variability of human response is remarkable. But just as the detective looks behind the obvious, picking up subtle clues, the therapist looks for the "soft signs" that add up to the hard indications of trauma.

If you get fooled in my business, it's usually because the patient appears to be better than he should be under the circumstances, not worse. The therapist must take into account not only the patient's particular situation but also her life history, what she says, and more significantly what she doesn't say. An adult-onset trauma that doesn't resolve as expected is often perched upon an underlying childhood trauma. The discovery of those underlying experiences means a more challenging treatment process.

Ella: A Child Is Murdered

When a parent has to face the death of a child, the wound can never be healed. When the loss is due to murder, the pain transcends agony.

There are support networks around the country for parents of murdered children, and my expanding work with EMDR trauma healing has guided me to involvement in this area. I had been awed by the work of Elaine Alvarez, an EMDR therapist and facilitator who had started the Inner Cities Project for an EMDR organization called Humanitarian Assistance Programs (HAP). The location I had chosen for my own EMDR work was the Bedford-Stuyvesant section of Brooklyn, since it was close to home and the residents were badly in need of help. Through a television program, I became aware of a group there called PURGE, whose members were mothers who had lost their children to gun violence. (An essential element in the trauma of a child's death is loss of choice and control. The sisterhood of PURGE helped alleviate that loss by initiating a landmark lawsuit against gun manufacturers. At least the women had the feeling that "there is something we can do.")

I hoped that forging a contact between HAP and PURGE could gain us trust and access in the community and pave the way for pro bono EMDR training of local Bed-Stuy therapists. Accordingly, I reached out to PURGE's cofounders, Yvonne Pope and Freddie Hamilton, two women whose courage has made them inspiring role models for me. Yvonne's son had been murdered two years earlier. She had already seen a therapist whom she felt could not relate to her suffering. When she told him her son's spirit had visited her after his death, the therapist had tried to persuade her that this had not happened. To her everlasting credit, Yvonne quit the treatment.

Yvonne ageed to try EMDR. We shared one ninety-minute session, during which her PTSD symptoms of flashbacks, hypervigilance, and irrational guilt eased dramatically. During the processing, she again experienced her son coming to her. She heard him say, "I'm okay now. I'll always be with you, watching over the family." This was a deeply healing experience for her and a profoundly moving one for me as well. A follow-up session reinforced her gains and carried her further in the recovery process.

These sessions convinced Yvonne of the power of EMDR. She invited my colleague Elaine Alvarez and me to a PURGE meeting one Saturday night in Bed-Stuy, to tell the other

members about EMDR. There were eight women at the meeting, and several expressed interest in how EMDR worked.
Elaine and I offered to give them a direct experience. Elaine
took one mother into a different room, but a powerful woman
named Ella, with pained, soulful eyes, opted to have a session in
front of the others; she said she wanted their support. I readily
agreed to her assertion of choice and control.

Five years previously, Ella's son Martin, a sixteen-year-old,
had been playing basketball with a group of friends, when he
was challenged by another boy who didn't like Martin's talking
to his girlfriend. The teen left, returned with a gun, and without warning at precisely 3:14 A.M. shot Martin dead. Ella was
immediately called and rushed to his side. She never had a
chance to say good-bye—he was already gone.

Ella started our session with the following challenge: "As a
man, you can never understand this. I feel like my umbilical
cord is still attached to Martin." Wearing headphones, Ella
went through bilateral stimulation, alternating between grief
and rage. All the images rushed past her: the call, hurrying to
Martin's side, his body covered with a sheet, his cold hand, the
sound of the ambulance that took him away, the funeral, the
days and months that followed.

Not once in the five years following the murder had Ella
fallen asleep before 3:14 A.M., the time Martin was shot. She
had to be at work by seven, so she was always sleep-deprived
and exhausted. At 3:13, she was awake; at 3:15 she was asleep. It
was unnerving, a fascinating symptom, demonstrating again
how biologically based symptoms are. In addition to scrupu-
lously processing all elements of the incident and its after-

effects, I also guided Ella to target this sleep problem. She was able to imagine herself falling asleep before 3:14. "I'll believe it when it happens," she reflected.

At the end of the session, she was amazed to find that images that had haunted her for so long had faded, their sting decreased. She thanked me for my effort and the group for their support. The other mothers, all of whom had lost sons (in some cases, more than one), seemed to have vicariously shared the healing experience.

Three days later Yvonne called me. Last night, she said, and the two nights preceding it, Ella had fallen asleep early and slept until morning. A follow-up six months later proclaimed similar results.

I left humbled by my contact with these brave women. How would I have stood up to a similar tragedy? I wondered. I was also haunted by their stories of mothers who had retreated to their houses following the death of a child, never to emerge again.

One year later we held our training for the community therapists of Bedford-Stuyvesant. Twenty-five therapists from community agencies were trained, and EMDR help is still being provided today to those who desperately need it. Similar trainings have been held in Newark, New Jersey, Washington, D.C., Oakland, California, and beyond.

And scores of suffering patients have received healing.

PHYSICAL TRAUMA

An auto accident is the most common kind of discrete trauma, and its effects on you will depend on a number of variables: whether you sustained an injury, and if so to what extent and how long it takes to heal; whether someone else got injured or killed, and your relation to that person; whether you were the driver or the passenger; whether the fault was yours or the other driver's. If a person is permanently disfigured in the crash, the extent of the healing from the trauma is somewhat limited. But despite the limitations to emotional healing—the very nature of the disfigurement will remain as a reminder of the accident—EMDR therapy *can* help.

Visual memory is an important component of most profound experiences. But in a car accident, sound (of the crash) and smell (of, say, gasoline) can leave a deeper imprint, which can be missed in therapy.

Recently I supervised an EMDR therapist who was treating a woman whose car had collided with a deer. She had survived with minor injuries, but her passenger, a close friend, had been killed. Therapist and patient had held multiple sessions, but the patient's SUDS level never fell below a 2.

"Did you process her through the image?" I asked.

"Yes."

"The sound?"

"Absolutely."

"The smell?"

"Oops. I forgot to ask." The therapist held another session with the woman. It was not the smell of gasoline that flashed back the trauma but the smell of the deer's blood. Once that smell was processed, the SUDS fell to 0. Again, this does not mean that the driver's grief at the death of her passenger disappeared; that loss was ongoing and abiding. Nothing could change that crushing reality. But EMDR therapy allowed its integration into the nervous system. What *did* vanish were the PTSD symptoms, in this case flashbacks (including smell), hypervigilance, and irrational guilt.

In processing a trauma that consisted of a mugging or a rape, the victim must overcome the remembered sensation of the bodily attack and often, in the case of a sexual assault, a powerful smell. The rape survivor's response to EMDR can be influenced by whether or not the rapist was apprehended, and where the attack occurred. But in all cases of brutalization, patients will exhibit a similar complement of symptoms: flashbacks, hypervigilance, nightmares, dissociative amnesia, and the like. As long as the incident remains stuck in the nervous system, no matter its cause, it will still be drawing from the same pool of symptoms and express itself in a universal way.

If in the real circumstances of her life the victim is now truly safe, the trauma tends to be simpler to resolve. If the perpetrator is caught, the belief that "it will definitely happen again" is clearly distorted. If the rapist remains at large, then the belief that "he will come back and get me" may be too strong, but it has some basis in fact. Unresolved situations impede a person's ability to fully accept that a traumatic incident is in the past, that he or she is safe and can go on now.

Claudia: Rollover on a Country Road

Claudia, a youthful, gregarious woman of fifty-seven, loved to drive. Her job as a legal assistant meant she had to travel from place to place in the upstate New York community where she lived and worked, but often she would just drive for pleasure, particularly on summer nights when the air was cool and the heavens brilliant with stars. Then four years ago her car, a two-door Nissan, was rear-ended on what she had thought was a deserted rural road.

The driver of the other car, a Corvette, was out-of-his-mind drunk. He was going ninety miles an hour when he hit the Nissan; there were no skid marks to indicate he had even attempted to avoid her. The Nissan rolled over four times, eventually coming to rest on its side, with Claudia trapped in the mangled metal. She blacked out briefly and woke up to an all-pervasive smell of gas. The motor was still running. Claudia, terrified, knew there was a good chance the car would ignite, yet it took her twenty minutes of mind-numbing effort simply to reach the ignition key. Even when she shut off the engine, she was almost choked by the smell, and not until an hour later, when the police were able to free her from the vehicle with the "Jaws of Life," was she able to breathe fresh air. The man who hit her was miraculously unhurt and had run off, leaving his car behind. He was easy to trace—a prominent, politically well-connected son of a local businessman—but he was never charged with a crime, not even drunken driving.

Claudia's injuries were serious: deep bruises, a broken leg, and a badly shattered arm. Still, her physical wounds healed quickly. It was to cure her emotional damage that, nine months later, she came to me.

We devoted the entire ninety minutes of our initial double

session to history-taking. She had old issues, as all of us do, but none seemed profound, and I knew it was primarily the trauma of the accident that we would target. For one thing, she could no longer drive by herself, and she was even uncomfortable when a friend drove her or when she went out at night.

Using EMDR, we began to process the accident. Most powerful for Claudia was the smell, then the feeling of rolling over, then the sound of the crash itself and of the running engine. Finally, there was the image of the broken windshield, which seemed to her to correspond to her own smashed body and shattered mind.

With bilateral stimulation, the patient gradually replays the image, as though running a movie in extraslow motion, virtually frame by frame. Then the images speed up. Claudia and I went over her images, from the crash through the arrival of the police to the paramedics rushing her to the hospital in the middle of the night. Issues arose over which friends and family members were there for her, and which were not. A key trauma centered on the fact that the other driver had escaped punishment—injustice is a common theme among trauma victims.

A week later Claudia returned for a second session. Her distress level had dropped from a 10 to a 4. I guided her through the sequence of the accident three times, once backward, an unusual approach I instinctively felt would help her. As always, I asked, "Would you like to try it?" and she readily agreed. At the session's end, her distress level was down to 0. Nevertheless, she still resisted getting back behind the wheel of a car and had to be driven by a friend.

No panic was involved in this resistance. Her brain—and this is common in trauma cases—couldn't comprehend that driving would be safe again, because it hadn't experienced it. A mock session, when I drew my chair alongside her to simulate driving, was not enough to break the impasse.

Sometimes therapists need to emerge from the safety of their offices, and this was one of them. I determined to become Claudia's "re-driving instructor," so I suggested she ask her friend if she could borrow her car.

Her friend drove to my office and left us the car. Claudia remained in the passenger seat, and I drove her to a deserted dead-end street. I gave her alternating vibrating tappers (called TheraTapper), which she slipped into her left and right shoes for bilateral stimulation; when we changed places, I made sure they would not get in her way when she actually drove. First, though, I guided her again through simulated driving.

"You ready to give it a try?" I asked.

She was a trouper. "Yes." Her voice was firm.

I knew there was a danger of her getting ahead of herself, so I instructed her to drive only to a car parked thirty feet ahead. "I don't want you to drive past it," I warned. Then I guided her to drive fifty feet. Then the entire block. More bilateral processing followed each positive experience.

Finally, near the end of our session, I told Claudia it was time to return to my office.

"I'll drive," she beamed.

I leaned back in the passenger seat. "Fine," I said. "You can drop me off in front of my building."

COMBAT TRAUMA

After World War I and World War II, many veterans returned with what was then labeled "shell shock" or "battle fatigue." Often they lived out their lives confined to VA hospitals or were afraid to leave home. These men had severe PTSD and might have been helped more if we knew then what we know now. Some are still alive and are restricted to hospitals. Case by case, I believe, the plights of some can still be eased.

The return of our Vietnam veterans, traumatized by a war we could not win, led to the designation of PTSD as a diagnostic category. The Vietnam War was unique. Trauma was intensified because the combatants followed few rules or conventions. It was terrifying to be in the jungle with its heat, snakes, mud, sounds, and smells, and the Vietcong exploited that terror as a conscious psychological weapon. GIs were captured and tortured, and their screams for help were used to draw comrades into the open, where they could be gunned down. Public displays of decapitated heads were common—on both sides. In Saigon women, children and the elderly who associated with you by day might become assassins at night. A state of alertness that would be deemed hypervigilance "stateside" was necessary for survival "in country." An otherwise beautiful paradise held unspeakable human atrocities. Both sides were witnesses to the depravity; both were left with crippled psyches, and haunted souls.

Had our soldiers returned as heroes, their trauma might have been less pronounced. Instead, forty-eight hours removed from a combat zone, they found themselves home with little or no debriefing, victimized by national denial and disregard. This only exacerbated the trauma symptoms, which were so severe that they were often misdiagnosed as psychosis.

I myself was not drafted due to a student deferment, but when I saw how I could help Vietnam veterans with PTSD, I began to seek them out. For me, helping these men and women was an honor. They had sacrificed so much; through EMDR, I could thank them.

TIM: SOLDIER OF MISFORTUNE

Tim came to me after every other treatment, psychopharmacological and psychiatric, individual and group, had failed. He had been labeled "uncooperative" by his therapists. He told me I was his "last hope," but, in truth, it seemed he had no hope.

Tim was the closest thing to a robot I'd ever seen. His facial expression was fixed, his body posture rigid, his voice without inflection. He spoke in a monotone. For me, it was both painful and frightening to experience him. He was of average size, not really menacing-looking, but his knowledge of how to kill—he seemed to relish shocking me by recounting the hundred different ways in minute detail—got my attention. At the end of each session, his eyes would lock into mine—and this guy had a *stare*.

"What are you doing?" I asked, when this first happened.

"I'm trying to look all the way to the back of your brain," he said.

Tim had spent nearly two years in Vietnam, almost all of them in combat, and now, twenty-eight years later, three-dimensional flashbacks of his experiences punctuated his every day. Flashbacks are not uncommon ("I can see it like it happened yesterday"), but Tim's were different. At any time, night or day, he was unwillingly propelled back to Vietnam. The heat, sights, smells, and sounds of jungle combat would envelop him, and he would be retraumatized again and again in a never-ending cycle of agony. He had been drafted at age twenty-seven, far later than most GIs. When he returned, little meaningful contact was possible between him and his family, supportive though they tried to be. He was lost in his own tangle of terrible sights and sounds.

Flashbacks were not Tim's only symptoms. Insomnia, headaches, intractable back pain, and difficulty breathing plagued him. Worse, however, was his crushing sense of guilt. He had been in a face-to-face standoff with a twelve-year-old boy when it was "kill or be killed." He chose to survive. He had "finished off" wounded enemies who were lying in the roadside and pleading to be spared, knowing how lethal they could be to him and his comrades. Once he had come across five GIs who had captured a Vietcong soldier and were torturing him to death. Repulsed, he nevertheless joined in, knowing they would turn on him if he refused. Tim's first goal was to come back alive—and he had. Yet he was haunted by his awareness of what he had done, and by his inability to forgive himself. He desperately needed my help, and I vowed to give him everything I could.

At first Tim was reluctant to share much of his experience with me, believing I might "turn him in" and he'd "face charges" because of his actions. But he gradually began to open up. He came to believe I would help him.

In my office, Tim was graphic and creative. One time he pointed to a knot low down in the wood of my doorframe. "The knothole's a bullet wound," he told me, "and the surrounding patterns are the blood coming out." He got on his hand and knees so he could trace the entry wound and the flow of blood. Any movie or documentary about war, even a depiction of the Crusades or the Roman conquests, triggered him. He told me that he'd often be up in the middle of the night, either because he couldn't fall asleep or because a nightmare had wakened him. Being with his own children heightened his grief at having killed children—indeed, he'd shot a teenage girl who, he swore, looked like his sixteen-year-old daughter, especially with her penchant for wearing black. He couldn't look at his daughter's face without the eyes of the Vietnamese girl staring back at him.

He had taken no pleasure in killing; he was just doing his job and staying alive the best way he could. We met for one ninety-minute session once a week, and slowly his traumatic symptoms started to unblock.

If images could wound, so could they heal. I asked him to consider all the enemy soldiers he had killed and then calculate how many lives he had possibly saved in so doing, instilling the idea of preserving life as well as taking it. For each person he killed, he calculated he had saved fifty lives, totaling five hundred GIs saved. I asked if he could imagine them gathering. Stimulated by the bilateral sound, he envisioned them in a VFW hall, safely home. At my suggestion, he visualized all the GIs' relatives filing into the hall, and soon he saw a room packed with people, alive and happy. This imagery, guided by me but conjured by him, represented a reality-based, concrete affirmation (rather than the abstract "I'm a valuable person"— something he struggled to accept). He imagined leading the GIs through the jungle to a clearing where a helicopter would take them to safety. This was a profound part of his healing, for it opened to him a pathway out of the jungle where he had literally been stuck.

With ongoing processing, the flashbacks went from 3D to flat; smell and sound also diminished, and the images would fade or go blurry. Some disappeared, some remained, and I wondered if Tim had suffered hippocampal shrinkage that could not be overcome. I held a joint session with him and his daughter, which helped him get closer to her, and actually walk with her by the ocean. The beach meant a good deal to him, and he told me that once, on R&R, he had gotten drunk and fallen asleep on the beach, awakening to find that a Vietnamese teenager was rifling his backpack. Many soldiers would have shot the boy on the spot, but this was not combat, and Tim simply chased him off. EMDR processing helped him integrate this caring act, as did befriending a Vietnamese orphan, whom he taught to read.

We were able to instill the belief that he was not a cold-blooded murderer deserving of hell, but a man capable of doing "the right thing." Not only was I nonjudgmental and supportive of Tim, but my genuine respect and admiration for his courage helped him feel worthwhile. He had fulfilled his goal in Vietnam of coming back alive. He did, and together we rediscovered together how positive a goal it had been.

We worked for a year and a half, and though we were never able to effect a 100 percent cure symptomatically, the 75 percent improvement was one of my greatest successes as an EMDR therapist. From the beginning I believed in Tim's capacity to heal with EMDR, although a team of therapists had already given up. He called me some six months ago to report on his progress. He had maintained emotional contact with his wife and children, and though at times he retreated, he always came back—sooner now than ever before.

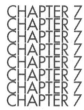

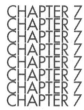CHAPTER 7 **GETTING UNSTUCK:**
HEALING TRAUMATIC EVENTS
FROM CHILDHOOD

Is any one form of childhood trauma "worse" than all others? The answer is complex. It depends on the victim's genetics, personality, and environment as well as the degree of trauma. Verbal abuse, for example, is a form of soul murder, and can be as bad as a beating; sometimes witnessing family violence (secondhand abuse) can damage a child as much as being the direct victim.

Sexual abuse tends to create the worst damage, even molestation short of penetration. But we can't compare human suffering; victims of verbal abuse and emotional abandonment also carry existential pain that may well demand attention from healers.

It's hard to know how far back into infancy we remember, though there have been documented instances of people remembering events that took place as early as three to six months. It's possible that we may even remember intrauterine experience, and Otto Rank has postulated that the experience of birth itself is a major trauma. Is it? I don't know. What we *can* know is that we remember through our symptoms. Panic attacks, depressed moods, rage reactions can all be feeling-state memories sheared off from the events that originally caused them.

When a patient is carrying childhood trauma, it will emerge relatively quickly with EMDR, unless it is buried under other layers of trauma. EMDR's powerful, direct access to the nervous system activates and reveals traumatic memories, as well as providing the vehicle to understand and heal them. It still amazes me that so much of a patient's processing is internal and rapid-fire, and that I never get to observe most of what leads to the incredible changes. Sometimes it's difficult for me to accept this loss of awareness and control. But it's an important reminder that healing potential lies almost entirely in the patient.

Ned: Trauma and the Reporter

Ned was a newspaper reporter on assignment in South Texas, covering border crossings by illegal immigrants. These men and women would try to enter the United States by fording the Rio Grande River, at times at its widest, deepest, and most turbulent section, and occasionally they would drown in the attempt. At one point in the river, there is an eddy that causes bodies to collect on the U.S. side, where Ned was often called to investigate. Sometimes, he'd spot fresh corpses in this section while driving to and from work.

I met Ned at a media conference in Texas, where the issue of occupational trauma came up. Ned had written his immigration stories a few years earlier and was still troubled by what he'd seen, but he downplayed the severity of his symptoms. In the reporting world, it's assumed journalists will be regularly exposed to nightmarish situations, and it is commonly accepted that they'll develop what a clinician would diagnose as PTSD symptoms. In effect, when reporters experience flashbacks, they assume they come with the territory and ignore them.

While Ned and I talked, he pointed out passionately that investigative reporters, like police officers, railroad engineers, and EMS technicians, regularly suffer trauma symptoms that they live with. I suggested he try EMDR, hoping that if it worked for Ned, he could pass word on to other reporters and let them know that a fast, effective treatment was available to them.

Ned readily agreed to try out a brief demonstration. His target image was of the eddy and the smell of the bodies, two different things, but to him they joined. His negative cognition was that "life is disposable," which is in some sense true, of course, but for him it had taken on a specific traumatic meaning. With the target image came the sound of swirling water. Ned had memories of field workers loading the bodies onto a truck and of sitting in his car as the truck passed, assaulting his senses with the odor of death. "It was an odor like no other," he told me. "Like nothing I've ever smelled before or since. It was beyond horrible." A sick look passed over his face. "Not only can I smell it, I can actually feel it, *taste* it in my throat now."

Smell can be the most powerful of our senses (a fact well known to perfume manufacturers), and this smell still gripped Ned years after the event. His distress level was high, at 8 or 9, and he felt burning anxiety in his throat, chest, and stomach. With EMDR processing, he flashed through an abundance of traumas he had experienced on the job. His SUDS level quickly dropped, but it stalled at 2. The image of the eddy faded but did not disappear; the smell was reduced but did not leave entirely.

Inexperienced EMDR therapists often think that in such a case, this must be as far as the client can go. But in fact, Ned's residual distress was really a diagnostic clue that there was more there, something as yet unrevealed. I asked him to let his mind drift back to his childhood, sensing that something related would emerge. Almost immediately his distress level spiked to a 6. He was suddenly five years old.

"The cat," he said. "We lived on a farm, a real rural, hard existence. One time the cat gave birth to a litter. I watched it. Then my dad came in and took the kittens and dropped them in a bag with some rocks and went down and tossed it in the creek." He shook his head. "It's funny. I hadn't remembered about those kittens until just this moment. Back then I thought I'd never forget it."

Ned's father's action demonstrated to the tender young boy that life was disposable. It was the silent underpinning of his adult negative cognition. He had no idea that these events were associated in his mind; the EMDR revealed it.

While processing the childhood memory, his SUDS level dropped to 0, and then he returned to the eddy. "Unbelievable!" His distress had vanished, and the sights and smells were gone. Only by locating and connecting with his early memory could he fully relieve the symptoms associated with the horrendous events at the drowning pool of the Rio Grande.

Ned's case reminded me of a patient named Isabelle, the twenty-year-old daughter of the former Peruvian ambassador to India. For years the sound of running water and a variety of smells, particularly of flowers, would trigger feelings of panic and obsessive thoughts of death in Isabelle. As a therapist, you have to have a sense when the fear of death is within appropriate limits, and when it is not, and in the case of a vital young woman like Isabelle, it was clearly excessive.

Using EMDR, she returned to the compound in India where her family lived when she was a toddler. The house abutted the Ganges. Isabelle suddenly recovered the sight of bodies floating down the river, festooned with flowers—the traditional Indian burial ceremony. At times her Indian nurse had lifted her to the window to watch at the ritual; it was considered beautiful in the nurse's culture. But long suppressed, it was this memory that lay behind Isabelle's terror and morbidity. Once discovered, the feelings vanished.

Ned's and Isabelle's cases both dealt with discrete traumas. More common in my practice is repeated childhood trauma.

RONNIE: THE FLIGHT OF THE CROW

Take one look at Ronnie, and you'd think, *Success.* Dressed in a Brooks Brothers suit, white button-down shirt, and conservative red tie, he looked like a forty-five-year-old midlevel executive in corporate America. He was, in fact, a dentist—and a successful one. But therapy revealed a mass of insecurities that had crippled him throughout his life. He needed help, he confessed to me. He was chronically depressed, limping through life, shackled by anxiety and dread. Nothing gave him pleasure. He could not feel good about himself, despite his high proficiency at his work. He had a stable marriage, and two wonderful children, but he was uncomfortable in their presence and was afraid his wife would leave him, taking the children with him. Years of prior therapy hadn't helped much. "It was like putting up curtains in my jail cell," he said.

I began, as always, by taking an extensive history.

Ronnie had been adopted at birth, taken into a family where there were already two natural children, Angie and Charlie, twelve and eight years older than their new baby brother.

Although most adoptive parents are loving and supportive, Ronnie's new mother was unstable and erratic in her behavior, loving one moment, verbally and physically abusive the next. The father was a passive, quiet man, unable to stem his wife's tirades or to protect the children against them. At times the mother would goad him into beating the children himself when he got home, further "punishment" for their "misdeeds."

Ronnie remembered most his mother's threats to "send him back to where he came from," though he had no idea where "back" was, only that it was someplace dark and unknown. As a ritual, she would pack his bags, drag him out to the car, and prepare to drive away; only his screams and promises to behave better would induce her to change her mind.

Ronnie's thoughts often drifted to fantasies of his birth mother, which led to guilt, and fear that the adoptive parents would retaliate by denying him love or throwing him out.

When Ronnie began EMDR treatment, the first memory to emerge was of his adoptive mother ushering him downstairs, carrying his bags toward the car. It elicited such terror even now, forty years later, that he felt electricity course through his body. We spent months processing this image and his belief, "My life is over." Gradually the terror was replaced by rage at being treated so cruelly, followed by sadness and grief over the suffering and lost years caused by his mother's emotional volatility.

Another image haunted him with equal power: a monstrous black crow. The image emerged repeatedly in dreams of a huge black bird flying in the house, swooping down, and pecking at him—terrorizing him. In processing the dream, he realized that there had in fact been a real crow, a real terror. His mother, who had a penchant for taking in stray animals and treating them with greater concern than she showed for her children, had kept a wild crow in a cage in the basement. Somehow it had developed the capacity to speak like a mynah bird. "Shut up! Shut up!" the crow would scream whenever Ronnie approached it. Its tone of voice echoed his mother's as well as the words, and his fear of the cellar soon matched his fear of being sent away.

The bird was filthy and emitted a putrid smell. Ronnie watched with horror as it grew too large for its cage and its beak twisted down against the bars until it could no longer open its mouth. In our sessions, he avoided the image for months, refusing to discuss it or to allow me to help him process it. But when he was finally ready to face it, processing quickly revealed that he identified with the bird. To him, the bird was a representation of himself: a foul animal, a foundling, worthless, trapped by his mother, imprisoned and tormented.

As described in Chapter 2, for EMDR to work to its potential, you have to locate a target image and develop a protocol around it. With discrete trauma, the target is right there and is usually quickly processed. With cases like Ronnie's, however, there are many targets, many images, many protocols. His case required eighteen months of intense work.

Beyond the stairs and the crow, I used two other major targets in Ronnie's treatment. The first had to do with his fantasies of his birth mother. His foster mother had told him that the woman was a prostitute, but in the course of treatment he came to understand that she wasn't; and that even if she had been, it didn't make her valueless. He sensed that for his birth mother, giving him up had been a profound loss, an insight that detoxified his adoptive mother's story of rejection.

The other major target involved his older sister, Angie, who had also been deprived of nurturance by her parents. When Ronnie was ten, she became physically seductive, inducing him into mutual genital stimulation. When an older male molests a girl, it is seen as sexual abuse; but when the situation is reversed, some believe it is the boy's "introduction" and say he is "lucky." This is simply false—sexual abuse is sexual abuse—and Ronnie was traumatized, for his arousal was mixed with intense guilt, shame, and fear. It took a long time for him to see that it was

Angie who was troubled, that he had done nothing wrong, that he was the victim, and that he was still suffering from the effects.

During the processing of his many protocols, which were resolved more and more quickly as the months went by, Ronnie passed through hundreds of different memories, all requiring some level of processing. In EMDR mourning is a crucial stage for patients to pass through in letting go of their traumas. A state that may appear to be regression is actually the patient's realization of the heavy toll and missed opportunities resulting from the trauma. The SUDS level may rise, but this actually presages letting go and moving on. If the therapist interrupts this grief work or doesn't support it, she risks retraumatizing the patient, denying his feelings and his losses. Once patients pass through their mourning stage and realize that grief is a natural consequence of the damage of trauma, they are ready to continue in the recovery process.

For Ronnie, the core issue was confusion about his identity. When his knowledge of who and what he was began to crystallize, his anxiety eased, his self-esteem rose, and his negative cognitions faded, replaced by positive cognitions such as "I have survived by my strength." He realized that his identity was the result of everything that had happened to him, good and bad, and that to deny what life had meted out to him was to deny himself. He was made up of his experiences, and he integrated them. Ronnie the crow opened his cage and escaped. Beating his strengthening wings, he soared above with a new perspective on the vistas below. After eighteen months of

EMDR treatment (as opposed to fifteen *years* of psychother-apy), he really believed he knew and felt good about himself. He began to highly value his work, using his gifts for potential changes he could make in the techniques of dentistry. He knew that his wife loved him and that he could openly show her love in return. He grew close to his children, no longer fearing he would hurt them or they him.

The real miracle of Ronnie's healing and recovery could occur only in the safety of the therapeutic relationship. As months went by, he came to trust me, to know that I was con-sistently accepting and available. He felt in control. The rela-tionship would end not by my throwing him out but by his choice, when he was ready. At the end, he knew there were more discoveries he could make about himself, but he felt that he had accomplished what he needed to. He knew he could come back if he wished, but he had met and exceeded his expectations, and this was his truth.

After a number of weeks, using EMDR to guide his separa-tion process, he opened my office door and flew off. My truth was that I was thrilled for his recovery but sad to see him go.

STELLA: PANIC AND THE PRIMAL SCENE

Sexual, physical, and verbal abuse are not the only lasting trau-mas children face. Sometimes they can be traumatized unwit-tingly by the ignorance or lack of awareness of their parents.

Stella, a meek, self-effacing woman in her mid-thirties, came to me at the recommendation of her doctor. She wore nondescript clothing, avoided eye contact, and spoke in a whisper, so that I had to strain at times to hear. An only child, she suffered from anxiety that had progressed to the point that she was unable to hold a job. She was claustrophobic; she panicked at the thought of being in a locked room. Elevators terrified her; when she was caught in a traffic jam, she wanted to flee; she feared driving over bridges and riding in a train. Eventually, these feelings had intensified to the point when she became agoraphobic. Through force of will, she could leave her house—generally to take her son to school—but it was torture for her, and at other times she had to be accompanied by a friend. When these symptoms last long enough, depression eventually sets in. (We call it secondary depression.) Stella felt hopeless and helpless, tangled up in her web of symptoms, crippled.

After three sessions of EMDR yielded little relief, I suggested that Stella be evaluated by a psychopharmacologist, for her symptoms were so unmanageable that successful treatment would take a very long time. The pharmacologist prescribed 20 milligrams daily of Prozac, a mild dose. Some might argue that the symptom reduction from the Prozac was all the help she needed; my sense was that it served to open the door to her therapy.

Help can come from the most unexpected places, as it did for Stella. When her husband, Andy, was driving her to her first session, he casually asked her, "Do you recall your earliest memory?" The question activated her, and it became the first target in our sessions. "I remembered lying in my crib," she told me, and suddenly tears streamed down her face. "I have no clue what's setting this off," she said.

She confessed an odd symptom that was especially striking. The sound of gum-chewing would sexually arouse her—confusingly, uncomfortably. It became acute if she was with her mother, but even when she was on a subway, the sound would disturb her and she would try to avoid it. Such strange symptoms leave a trail for therapeutic detective work, and they often lead to a traumatic experience hidden away by dissociation.

We couldn't start with a full EMDR protocol; although the crib imagery evoked grief, it was too abstract to provide any negative cognitions. Gradually, though, session by session, the scenario filled out. The thought "I'm trapped" emerged for her, along with a precipitous jump in her anxiety level.

The crib was in Stella's parents' bedroom (information she was able to corroborate), and her memory was of lying there, stock-still, immobilized by terror as she heard the noise of her parents making love. She was trapped in the room, in a crib, afraid to look over or let out a peep. The immobilization was psychological as well as physical. Her tears in my office, she came to realize, stemmed from the fact that there was something deeply painful in the memory.

We processed this initial target for nine months, during which time countless memories, some seemingly meaningful, some not, crossed her mind. She remembered her terror when, at age five, she had first learned to read and saw a newspaper headline that a woman had been attacked. One time she brought up the image of her father's disabled sister who had come to visit one day—and the next day died during a grand mal seizure.

Through it all, Stella continually cycled back to the sound of gum-chewing. She was embarrassed to bring it up, reluctant to speak about it. "I can't believe I'll be saying things to you I wouldn't say to my husband," she whispered—and then she'd tell me.

Her image was of oral sex, of her father putting on a condom, followed by her mother chewing it off his penis. This may have been a condensation of two separate acts—putting on a condom and oral sex; whatever, it was accompanied by the smell of sex—chewing and sex combined.

She realized that her current panic was the same as the terror she had felt in her early years, literally trapped in her crib, when she knew something was happening but didn't know what. Her images moved ahead chronologically (a key sign of healing in the EMDR process), as she stayed in her parents' bedroom until she was five. She had been exposed to the primal scene countless times, and she integrated it into every developmental step of her early childhood.

We kept returning to the crib. The image continually changed as she reexperienced feeling trapped in her parents' bedroom progressively from ages one to five. It would have been an error to use EMDR to desensitize her panic without ferreting out its root causes. It's far better to access the source of the symptoms than to try to relieve the symptoms first. In Stella's case, the accessing and processing of the source of her symptoms yielded change not only in connecting with the past but in behavior evident in the present. Gradually, she came out of her shell. She could maintain eye contact and project herself in a full voice. Her clothes became more stylish and feminine. Her panic abated, and her depression vanished. She was able to separate emotionally from her daughter and began substitute teaching. Although her fear of confinement was gone, her avoidance of closed places continued. Some symptoms die hard.

I believed she could face closed places without fear but held back from saying so. "It's your choice," I told her, "but I'm going to suggest we take an elevator ride together. You can even wear the headphones and listen to the sounds." My office is on the second floor of a three-story building, and she had always walked up the stairs to reach it. Although avoidance was her habit, I offered her both encouragement and choices, and she reluctantly agreed to the experiment. We took the elevator up and down several times, then returned to my office.

"How was that?" I asked.

"I didn't like it."

"What about your anxiety?"

"I didn't have any."

Illogic is not uncommon in recovering from trauma. Like many others, Stella felt lost without the panic that had been with her for decades: "Who will I be without it?" Gradually she confronted her panic on her own; one by one the dominoes of fear fell. First she took the train to the city with her daughter, then followed up by taking the same ride by herself. Her successes were reinforced with bilateral stimulation. Next she was able to drive across the Whitestone Bridge. She lost her way but recovered, then got stuck in a traffic jam, but neither time did she panic. But such journeys still didn't "feel right" to her and each trip generated uncovered memories, indicating that her trauma had yet to be fully processed.

Over the course of the next twenty-four months, the memories of being trapped in her crib in her parents' bedroom faded away in stages. Gradually the sound of chewing gum did not trigger a response in her. She was able to go off the Prozac, which led to a temporary upswing in anxiety, which we retargeted and processed through. And then one day a new image emerged. She was again in her parents' bedroom, but this time she was out of the crib. She was on her feet, and she turned from the sight of the bed, walked to the door, and left the room, closing the door firmly—and forever—behind her.

JIM: ESCAPE FROM THE PIT

Childhood trauma comes in many forms. As a boy, Jim was not abused himself, but his father's continual abuse of his mother— mostly verbal, but occasionally physical—was as damaging as if Jim himself had been the recipient of the blows.

Jim, at twenty-nine, was six foot five, 240 pounds, yet when I first saw him, he seemed much smaller. His shoulders were stooped, his head was bowed, and his eyes were downcast, as though afraid to face me, let alone the world. Yet he was a self-made man. He had developed his computer expertise into a successful consulting business; he had been able to use his talent and drive successfully in this unconflicted area of his life.

His problems were in relationships. He could not handle rejection by a woman. Frightened of abandonment, the slightest real or imagined criticism from a girlfriend would trigger a torrent of yelling, ending in despair. Exaggerated anger is often a clue to the presence of a trauma history. The first signs of impending rage are usually experienced bodily ("I feel my chest tightening" or "My head feels like it's going to explode"). These body sensations are often visceral memories of early traumas, and processing them has the dual effect of opening up new material and defusing the explosiveness.

Jim came to see me because he had just broken up with his girlfriend of six months. He had decided to take a week's vacation surfing in Hawaii with a few of his male friends, and she had complained that he should have spent the time with her. She expressed her hurt and anger—they were appropriate feelings, which she communicated appropriately—and he snapped and became abusive. "Once I got rolling," he said, "I couldn't stop. It happens all the time." In the aftermath of this exchange, he spiraled down into what he called "the pit."

We processed several specific memories with EMDR: his father's abuse of his mother; his mother's retaliation, sometimes at him, sometimes at Jim's brother; his father's death when Jim was fourteen. Shortly thereafter, Jim began to abuse alcohol to ease his pain, a period that lasted seven years. Desperate, he attended an AA meeting and his recovery began; he's been sober for seven years. (Alcoholism has a clear genetic and biochemical aspect, although environment and identification are powerful factors as well. I have never met an alcoholic or anyone wrestling with addiction who did not carry a strong trauma history, often the effects of growing up in an alcoholic family. The addiction itself, with all the damaging experiences it leads to, becomes a new trauma on its own. I have found that EMDR, with its potent ability to heal trauma, can be extremely helpful in supporting the recovery from addiction, even in helping to reduce the cravings that grip the body.)

We targeted Jim's father's death and many of the incidents of his own alcoholism, but in our sessions he'd see looming before him the depressed, angry, disapproving face of his mother—and again he would descend into "the pit." Although I encouraged him to see the pit as a good target for EMDR processing, he pulled back. "I don't want to go anywhere near it. It will swallow me up."

It took several months to help Jim understand that the only way to escape his demons was to face them—a technique similar to "flooding," used in behavior therapy to desensitize phobias, in which you help the patient learn by experience that the problem is the fear alone, not the situation itself.

"Tell me about the pit," I asked.

"It's fifteen feet deep, four feet across, dark, muddy and dank."

"Where are you now?"

His face contorted. "I'm in the pit. It's filthy."

"What happens when you look up?"

"I see the sky up there. But I'm trapped. I'll never get out."

The pit felt real to him, although it was only a metaphor. He was trapped in his fear and guilt, holdovers from the self-blame, terror, and childhood experiences of being helpless in an abusive, alcoholic family where misery was a daily experience for all. He had vivid memories of himself as a young boy waiting in suspense for calamity to happen; usually it did, which only added to the fear. He couldn't shake the belief that if he had been a better child, things wouldn't have been so bad. His home life was indeed like living in a pit.

During processing he often became scared, angry, sad, hopeless, and despairing of any change. At one point the pit filled with murky water, and he felt he would drown. At another he could see his parents looking over the rim, their faces filled with scorn. Then the sky would grow so dark, he couldn't see out at all. He experienced a variety of body sensations—heaviness in his chest, shoulder pain, pressure in his head—but with great courage he'd face the pit in session after session, and he'd stay with it for as long as he could.

Finally, rays of sunlight came from above. The pit got smaller. He could see himself emerge. Then he took the ghosts of his scorning parents, threw them into the pit, and covered them over. But they were powerful. He'd see their hands emerge, clutching at him, trying to pull him back in.

Still, he edged farther and farther away from the pit until one day, spontaneously, he realized that "the pit was inside me." With the awareness that the pit was internal rather than external came an equally startling epiphany. He had used the past tense: The pit *was* inside him. It was no longer there now. Further processing strengthened his grip on this newfound concept. Near the end of his EMDR sessions, he was startled by another realization: "There were good times in my family. We used to laugh a lot." This was followed by, "You know, I got some good things from my folks. I had to. Look at what I've been able to do with my life."

Today, Jim has less and less fear of relationships. Not only is he able to communicate his own negative emotions, he has learned to do so in a constructive manner. He still has occasional flare-ups of temper and sadness, but he catches himself quickly. He is in a healthy relationship now. He and his girlfriend had an argument the other evening, he told me, but made up and didn't go to bed angry.

We try to associate the word *normal* with ourselves, but it never quite seems to fit. Most of us hold to the social contract of *pretending* to be normal, but inside we're struggling with a variety of "crazy" or "twisted" fantasies and behaviors that we try to keep hidden. No one knows this better than therapists. In working with thousands of people, I've encountered amazing stories of love and hate, tragedy and triumph. Each one is fascinating and inspiring. My patients afford me the privilege of peering into the windows of their soul. And usually the clearest window lies not in the mind but in the body.

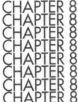

CHAPTER 8 EMDR AND THE BODY

EMDR is essentially a body-oriented treatment. The purpose
of the step-by-step protocol, proceeding from target image to
cognition to emotions, is to arrive at the container of the body.
Once the patient has reprocessed an experience, the final step
validating the completion of the healing is to scan the body. Is
there any tension left? Any discomfort or uneasiness?

A newborn baby cannot differentiate between body sensation and emotion. Hunger, being soiled, fear, frustration, and
contentment are all felt in the body and are differentiated only
as comfort and discomfort. The reptilian brain and the body are
acting as one. Discomfort is discomfort, whether it's emotional
or physical. The same thing applies to comfort.

BRAIN, MIND, EMOTION—AND BODY

It's absurd to talk about the mind without talking about the
body. Emotions, impulses, thoughts, and desires all are fully

integrated in the body and cannot be experienced without the body's participation. Many forms of psychotherapeutic treatment recognize this principle and use biochemistry to go right at the body without the "intervention" of talk. By contrast, psychoanalysis is devoted primarily to verbal interchange, using the patient's reported dreams and stream of consciousness to access the conflicts, fears, and childhood experiences that underlie troubled behavior.

EMDR itself is centrally located among the various forms of psychotherapy. If you imagine a wheel with all other psychotherapies as its spokes, EMDR can be found at its core. Thought, sensory memory, emotion, and body experience are all components of psychological life and cannot be separated. If you ignore the body in trying to understand emotion, you lose the resonance of the feeling. How we demonstrate our emotions through posture, facial expression, and "body language" is as crucial to communication as spoken words. No social contact, no intimate relationship, no business exchange exists without body language. For it is here that the unconscious, unspoken, underlying feelings are expressed. "I love you," the young woman says to her boyfriend, shying away from his touch. "I won't hurt you," the bully promises, aggressively in his victim's face. "That's my best offer," the salesman says, suddenly sweating, pupils dilating. In each case, it is the language of the body, not the words surrounding it, that speaks the truth.

EMDR presents constant opportunities to access meaning through the body and in some instances to treat emotions that are preverbal. If, at three months, a baby falls into a pool and

nearly drowns, that trauma is recalled in the sensation of suffo-
cation along with the terror that accompanied it. Years later it
might show up as a breathing difficulty, perhaps asthma or
panic attacks. Experiences that are reminiscent of the original
trauma will trigger an adrenaline release by the brain that is felt
primarily in the body. From brain to body to brain is a loop
that has no true beginning or end.

PHYSICAL CONDITIONS

Physical ailments always have an accompanying overlay of
emotions. Heart disease, for example, will often trigger a
depressive or panicky response. Loss of function or health can
dent or even shatter your sense of self or your faith in life. From
birth, we subconsciously know how our bodies work: blood
flow, breathing, digestion, hormonal release. This existential
experience is of our bodies from the inside out and the outside
in, yet our thinking processes do not usually register it unless
something goes wrong—breathlessness, chest pains, a scrape or
a cut.

Body sensations are a form of visceral communication that
yields rich information when processed with bilateral stimulation. "I feel a knot in my stomach," the patient says. "Go from
there," the therapist replies. "See where your mind takes you."
The feeling—a clenched stomach—is a common one and can
hold many meanings. The idea of a *knot* being there can be rep-
resentational—the patient might have been tied up in his
childhood, or even beaten with rope—or it can be completely

figurative, without direct symbolic significance. Sometimes it falls in between. In the case of a patient prone to anxiety, the therapist may wonder why the sensation is described as a "knot" rather than a "burning fire," "lead weight" or "knife." At times the mystery unfolds and clues are revealed; at other times they remain obscured.

"There's a heaviness on my shoulders," a patient reflects. Process the experience, and the patient may remember being pushed or held down as a child. Or the memory may simply be pressure from an overbearing parent. The body speaks in sensory metaphor; during EMDR the mind is helped to interpret it; the memory is integrated in thought and emotion. And healing is within reach.

EMOTIONS AND THE BODY

Since everything in the mind affects the body and everything in the body affects the mind, I believe that the currently popular term *mind-body connection* is misleading. Mind and body are one. A far better description is *the system,* which connotes the idea of integration and flow, where flow is the expression of emotion.

People carrying emotional burdens will usually feel them bodily, although the body can dissociate from physical sensations the way that the mind does with emotions. Depression is often accompanied by sensations of heaviness and feeling slowed down. Anxiety brings on a tightening in the chest, a burning in the stomach, or back pains. PTSD yields hypervigilance and sensitivity to sounds and smells associated with the trauma.

There's no line between the effect of trauma on the mind and on the body. Nevertheless, body is sometimes "only" body, and any reasonable psychotherapist will make sure that body symptoms are checked out first to determine if the symptoms have a physical basis. These days a classic error that a few therapists make is to blindly treat physical symptoms as psychological in origin.

When therapists treat physical conditions as though they were emotional ones, at best they are misinterpreting the message the patients are communicating; at worst, they are putting the patients at risk. I've worked with individuals who presented classic panic symptoms, yet medical tests showed physiological problems such as respiratory or thyroid dysfunction. I had them seek appropriate medical treatment before attempting to determine if psychological treatment was necessary.

When body sensations processed with EMDR vanish and do not return, this diagnostically suggests (but does not prove) that the symptom was psychosomatic in origin. And if the symptom doesn't move, or comes back quickly after psychological treatment, then the chances are greater that the symptom is physical and needs medical treatment, or that the emotional issues are extremely deep-seated and complicated.

JOAN: ASTHMA AND THE SPIDER

The way in which the body manifests PTSD—and the challenge of discovering whether a condition is physical or psychosomatic—was demonstrated by a recent patient of mine.

Joan is twenty-six. Six years ago her father was run down by a car and killed instantly in front of Joan's house. From the kitchen, Joan heard the sound of the car's brakes and the collision with the body and rushed outside—to find her father lying in the roadway. He had sustained massive, fatal internal injuries, but to Joan he seemed merely asleep.

Joan handled the situation with amazing presence of mind, calling 911 and speaking coherently to the police. But perhaps she handled it "too" well. Within a week of the accident, she developed asthma for the first time in her life.

Asthma may appear to be an emotionally derived condition, yet all medical tests suggest it is physical in origin. Did Joan have a predisposition to it? Possibly. Was it a preclinical condition? Perhaps. Yet as we were processing the image of her father in the street and the sound of the impact, she became acutely asthmatic and struggled to breathe.

With her permission, I followed my instinct and gently applied pressure to her hands, alternating between left and right. Perhaps the physical contact would help ground her, I thought. I asked her to image her asthma experience.

"I have a huge spider in my chest." (She later shared that she had visualized this image many times over.)

As we used this tactile version of EMDR, she imagined the spider starting to crawl up her throat, and her agitation increased. I slowed down the process and spoke soothingly to her: "What are you feeling now?" "It's crawling up higher." Her processing stayed with this image as the spider crawled up her throat and into her mouth. She then imagined spitting it out on the floor, where at last she squashed it with her foot.

Its expulsion and destruction were a tremendous relief as

well as a great surprise. Joan reported that she physically felt 90 percent better, but a rawness remained in her chest. We processed this, and quickly the sensation disappeared when she imagined a cool blue liquid coating her lungs. Could it have been that her asthma was a symptom of PTSD and that the spider was symbolic of the fact that her father's unseen injuries were internal? It's hard to say for sure. But, as of this writing, she has had no recurrence of the symptoms. I believe that without EMDR she would still be having them. Will they come back at a later time on their own, or perhaps be triggered by a new traumatic experience? Only time will tell.

DISSOCIATION

The dissociation of trauma memories and their attendant emotions frequently leads to altered bodily experiences. Some people may feel as if some part of them is missing ("I can only feel myself from the waist up"), while others may experience a variety of strange sensations. An anorexic distorts her body image, believing she is fat, resulting in self-starving behavior. A bulimic blocks her emotional pain with almost addictive food bingeing and purging.

Body dysmorphia, the feeling that one part is too large or too small or unusually ugly (a nose, for example), is another dissociative phenomenon. For example, a patient of mine felt that her hair was disgusting to the sight and touch. In fact, her blond hair was a striking aspect of her overall beauty, but her abusive mother had always denigrated her hair as being "too fine" (a comment many would take as a compliment). When we targeted this symptom with EMDR, the memories that lay behind it emerged, and the woman remembered countless incidents where her mother had beaten her and called her a "disgusting tramp," starting when she was three years old. Her symptom both covered and expressed her traumas that assaulted her sexuality and core sense of self. One year of regular EMDR sessions released her from her traumas and confusing, crippling symptoms.

Hair is certainly an issue for men, but in John's case it went beyond all logic. He was a good-looking man with long hair tied back in a ponytail. "Women found it sexy," he told me. But when his hairline started to recede, his reaction was intense. Mortification, depression, and an inescapable feeling of unattractiveness led him to wear hats, even indoors. ("Women don't find me sexy anymore.") Our history-taking yielded memories of his father beating John on the head when he was a little boy. EMDR targeting of his traumas revealed that his symptom was both literal and symbolic of the assault on his masculinity. John realized he was projecting his own distorted beliefs onto the women he dated, thereby compounding his misery. After fifteen sessions of targeting his memories with EMDR, we turned to what remained of his distorted beliefs. In two sessions they were gone and treatment was complete.

CONNECTIONS

Reptiles function well with their reptilian brains. Mammals adapt well to their environments with their reptilian and mammalian brains. We human beings, with the addition of our thinking brains, have lost much of our animal instinct, complicating our relationship with our bodies. In other words, our greatest asset as people is also our greatest deficit as members of the animal kingdom.

If a river otter is raised in captivity and at one year of age is released into its natural environment, it adapts immediately. Try the same experiment with a chimpanzee, however, and it can't survive. The higher up we go on the phylogenic scale—the more advanced our brains become—the more distant is our connection to our bodies. It's the price we pay.

Adaptation results from making connections neurophysiologically, and people who have trouble adapting struggle to make these connections. The belief "I can't do it" is often systematically held. ("I can't attract women because my hair is falling out," "I can't survive on my own"), and too often the belief becomes self-fulfilling. EMDR helps people regain the connections that were broken or blocked by traumatic experience. It fosters connections between the different parts of the brain and the body within the system as a whole.

ENHANCEMENTS

The final step in the setup of the EMDR protocol is locating the body sensations. This is followed by the application of bilateral stimulation and the beginning of the EMDR processing. There is value in repeatedly checking in with the body *throughout* the sessions, bringing the patient back to the body experience, asking what imagery the body sensations evokes. A therapist may ask: What would you imagine the sensation looks like? What is its color, size, shape, weight, temperature? (Color activates many areas in the brain as well as carrying symbolic meaning.) What starts as a black anvil, say, on someone's shoulders can morph into a rod of gray metal, then become a half-dollar. How can these changes be described neurologically and psychologically? We don't really know.

In the face of negative body sensations, I find it helpful to identify the positive feelings in the body. I ask the patient to tell me not only about tension and discomfort but also where he or she feels bodily clear, relaxed, and comfortable. Aware of a heavy feeling in the chest, a patient will be surprised to find that his legs are relaxed. By accessing positive sensations and using bilateral sound stimulation, the feeling often spreads. The body becomes an agent for access to negative *and* positive feelings, to the patient's full range of neurophysiological, psychological, and spiritual resources. Identifying the positive in the presence of the negative helps patients see that they have resources even while experiencing vulnerability both emotionally and bodily.

Psychotherapy, by definition, means healing of the mind. Yet Freud himself started as a neurologist and recognized the body's importance, identifying that we go through oral, anal, and phallic phases, though for him the ultimate solutions lay in the brain. In EMDR, an integrative therapy, the body is a core aspect of healing.

When we think of ourselves, we usually don't think in terms

of body. We echo Descartes: "I think therefore I am." But our bodies are ourselves, every bit as much as our thoughts and emotions.

Most of what we are does not reside in the forebrain; the cortical brain only caps off everything that lies beneath. We are physical beings, shaped by sexuality and aggression. To express emotions through making love, we need to touch and be touched. It is the most profound way to express that most meaningful feeling, although abuse and shame can pollute it. Sexuality can bring us together or drive us apart. When intertwined with aggression, it can emerge as sadomasochism, rape, and sexual abuse. These reflect our neurophysiology gone awry, distortions of the mind/body system.

IN SUM

Trauma is part of the human experience and affects all aspects of the human system. EMDR is an integrative approach to healing that system. It identifies and activates the trauma held in the system and then releases it. Use of the protocol (and its variations) combined with bilateral stimulation culminates in the body and brings about the comprehensive effects of EMDR, which by its nature heals systemically. Those of us who are therapists have little direct influence over our patients' internal process, which they essentially experience bodily. As we structure the protocol, our wisdom is to recognize this physical truth and to work within its context.

Healing a patient's trauma is impossible without healing the whole system, physiologically, neurobiologically, and psychologically. The arm doesn't function independently from the leg; similarly, emotions and thoughts don't flow in a different system from the body. EMDR is an integrative approach to an integrated system that is centered in the body. And, as we shall see in the next chapters, two essential elements of this system which supports us are performance and creativity—vital aspects of healing and of life.

III
ALL THE WORLD'S A STAGE: EMDR AND PERFORMANCE ENHANCEMENT

CHAPTER 9
CHAPTER 9
CHAPTER 9
CHAPTER 9
CHAPTER 9
CHAPTER 9
CHAPTER 9
CHAPTER 9 **THE BEST THAT YOU CAN BE**

To a great extent, the enhancement of performance—athletic, artistic, oratorical, professional, social, personal, and in relationships—lies outside the realm of psychopathology and trauma. But not entirely. performance blocks are often trauma related, although not necessarily in a direct one-to-one connection with a particular activity.

No one goes trauma-free during the course of life. Saying you've never been traumatized is like saying you have a defect-free body, ignoring genetics, illness, injury, and the aging process. Moreover, trauma affects all aspects of the person, yet there are experts who work with performance enhancement—some sports psychologists—who don't address past traumas that reside in an individual's neurophysiological system, limiting their focus to present emotional and thinking processes instead. This can limit their work's effectiveness, much like cutting down weeds but leaving the roots to grow back.

Our performance is most often impeded by the distorted

beliefs we hold about ourselves, often unconsciously. When we project these distorted assessments into the world, we become convinced that others—our "audience"—see us in the same critical way. These negative self-assessments pervade our entire *systems,* distorting our images of ourselves and of others. But as we are not mind-readers, we rarely know what others think of us. Those who suffer from social anxiety and are terrified by attending parties are a good example: they actually elevate their importance by putting themselves in a critical spotlight of their own irrational invention. In reality, most people are too concerned with how they themselves are coming across to focus such inflated attention on someone else.

Performance is intertwined with perception, whether it is accurate or distorted. When we project our own negative perceptions onto those observing us, we activate our anxiety, shame, and inhibition, undermining our performance. When we view ourselves positively, our performance is enhanced.

And performance is an everyday, all-day experience. It doesn't matter whether we're driving on a highway, answering a question in a classroom, socializing, telling a joke at a party, or even folding an envelope in a post office—"all the world's a stage." Even at the highest levels of performance (acting Hamlet, pitching in major league baseball), people are still dealing with basic human issues: success and failure, competition, achievement.

A few sports psychologists tend to work only with positive visualization, relaxation exercises, and affirmations. Such techniques are valuable in a limited context, but they miss the point that a performer has a system shaped by history: what you put in is what you get out; the nature of the solution is defined by the nature of the problem. Resolving problems only on the surface leads to superficial adaptation, not resolution. And these adaptations tend to be limited in duration—the problem will likely reassert itself later or emerge in another form.

Performance is in the now, in the moment. Bill Russell, a great basketball star of the 1950s and 1960s, describes the moment in which all outside factors in the game—the crowd, body pain, even the score—vanish, and he is one with the flow of the action. It is a sublime moment, he says, when winning or losing are meaningless. It is a fusion of body and spirit, of instinct and skill, of rehearsal and spontaneity. I've had similar experiences with public speaking (an act of which I was once terrified), when I am connected with my audience, when my thoughts and words flow effortlessly, when I am aware that I am expressing my thoughts at the peak of my ability. In that moment, I lose consciousness of everything save the fact that I'm doing what I should be doing, that I'm the best I can be in that moment.

People suffering from depression often live in the past, while people overwhelmed with anxiety live in the future. EMDR brings a person fully to the present. Therapy works as a process when patient and therapist are *both* in the moment, where the highest level of truth is not then or when but now.

PERFORMANCE BLOCKS

Have you ever walked into a meeting with strangers and felt that everybody was looking at you? Have you ever experienced a sudden drop of self-confidence at a job interview or when speaking in public? Have you ever felt in any situation, professional or social, that you're inadequate or a fraud, that "they can see right through me"?

These beliefs, and others like them, inhibit performance. Sometimes people blind themselves with grandiosity—for example, the atonal karaoke singer who's convinced she sounds like Barbra Streisand, or the self-delusional Casanova blind to his beer belly and receding hairline. But far more common is a sense of fraudulence—the feeling that "I'm not good enough (not the right person) to be doing what I'm doing." The woman at the party who feels that everybody's looking at her, that she's over- or underdressed and her makeup is off, that she's going to say the wrong thing and make a fool of herself is projecting her distorted image of herself. For chances are she's presentable, and what she has to say is interesting enough.

Social phobia is an intense version of shyness, sometimes so crippling that it even prevents its sufferers from attending dinners with friends. Targeted bilateral stimulation is an effective tool in getting to its root causes, as it is in finding the source of all performance inhibitors. For social phobia doesn't arise out of nowhere, but from experiences when facing the world earlier in life; its severity depends on the degree of those negative experiences.

To resolve a client's performance anxiety effectively, even to remove a single specific block, the therapist needs to explore the client's personal history. He may have to look into painful experiences from the past to ease away the block, and that process may be unsettling. EMDR locates root causes at warp speed, helping the client discover parallels between past events and present performance difficulties. The client quickly sees that these connections are held in his own system.

ARNOLD: ECHOES AND SPEAKING ANXIETY

Those who suffer from fear of public speaking describe their anguish as worse even than the fear of death. As Jerry Seinfeld describes it, "At a funeral most of us would rather be in the box than delivering the eulogy."

Arnold, at forty-six, is a highly successful, highly accomplished business executive, head of a medium-sized public relations firm. He does brilliant work on his own and has won several awards for his marketing programs. But at meetings, especially with strangers, when he has to "sell" his ideas, he panics and locks up. "I don't know my stuff," he worries. "I'll make a major mistake. Cost my company. Damage my position." No amount of reassurance helps, either from his family (he is happily married with two teenage sons), or from his colleagues. When the panic attacks became so severe he could only croak out his presentations, he sought me out.

Arnold began by processing the protocol. In *five seconds,* he heard echoes of his father's voice: "Shut up, stupid!" it told him. "You can't get anything right. *You don't know what you're talking about!"*

There it was. Warp speed.

Once this connection was made, Arnold's memories went

back to the time at age three, when he first remembered hearing his father's derision, and then he flashed through countless childhood memories. His father was verbally abusive to his mother and sister, particularly his mother, while Arnold would cringe and wonder why his mother didn't defend herself.

Arnold processed more early experiences, and as he traveled back and forth from past to present, the correlation between his father's abuse and his own terror became clearer and clearer. You might wonder why he had never made the connection himself—it seems obvious as I present it here. But he had been traumatized, leading to dissociation and disconnection. It took EMDR to reestablish the connection, and once it did so, his life changed. He still felt mild anxiety at public meetings, but the panic was gone and he was able to present his ideas with a clear voice and a clear mind. He could have gone deeper and learned more, but relief from his terror was all he wanted, and I did not push him. What he had discovered was how deep the roots of his panic ran.

EARLY LIFE EXPERIENCE

The first performance in life is birth (or perhaps it's conception). Otto Rank postulated that birth itself is traumatic, and enough people seem to have made the connection between birth trauma and later life experience to lend support to the theory. In my own case, I underwent a difficult birth, arriving with my umbilical cord wrapped around my neck. Did this account for the feelings and images of asphyxiation that flashed through my head in my own first EMDR session? Maybe yes, maybe no. But I wouldn't deny the possibility.

A baby smiles. Rolls over. Crawls. Begins to walk. How the caretaker responds to her is crucial to developing her confidence and sense of self. Does the child receive mirroring of her developmental accomplishments? ("Look at what baby did!" the mother exclaims, smiling back.) Or does she receive criticism? ("You always mess things up.") Or perhaps most damaging, does she receive apathy? ("You're not even worth noticing.") Such negative responses, if repeated habitually, will be internalized, and the child will play them out later socially with other children, in day care, in kindergarten. And a pattern of "bad" behavior, temper outbursts, "acting out," sullenness, and so on, will develop. This will lead to more negative mirroring from teachers and peers and will only deepen the child's negative self image and poor performance.

These traumas form the foundations of negative self-perception and behavior in adult life. Few performance experts speak of the impact of these experiences, but they go directly to the core of an individual's success or failure. Public performance and social interaction involve the basic issue of trust, which begins at infancy.

WORKING WITH CELEBRITIES

For people in the public eye—actors, athletes, politicians, writers, artists, musicians, entertainers—performance issues are exacerbated, since celebrities face different situations from the rest of us. Among other things, they are treated as commodities. Many of them were child prodigies, valued less for who they were than for what they did or produced, and thus they became dissociated from their core being. Their gifts led to their exploitation through commercialization, socialization, and adulation, and it became difficult for them to hold on to their sense of self. (This is why so many celebrities speak of themselves in the third person or adopt stage names.)

We look at celebrities not as people but as embodiments of our own fantasies. ("We won!" we exult when the team we support clinches a championship.) But our projections have little or nothing to do with them as people; they are our own idealized reflections, meant to satisfy our own unmet needs. The repeated denial of who you truly are is a profound form of emotional abandonment.

The "special treatment" that celebrities receive can itself be damaging. For instance, I've heard stories of celebrities receiving *inferior* medical care from stargazing medical professionals who could not insist on the same compliance to treatment that they would require of all their other patients. Such modified care is another form of retraumatization, like the childhood abandonment, familiar to the star by now, ignoring their needs and essential vulnerability.

With the famous, the therapist must remain the confident expert, just as he is with anybody else. Performers may be defensive ("I can handle it—I'm a *star*"), or they may be arbitrarily late or miss appointments, thus undermining their own progress. Many resent and are threatened by authority figures because as prodigies they lost their youth and are therefore mistrustful of adults. But the therapist must hang in there, resolutely committing to the person's healing.

With EMDR, which is based on structured set of protocols and procedures, the therapist has to assert his "parental" limit, resisting the celebrity's seductions such as "Why do I have to do it this way?" or "Why can't I talk out my problems like I did with all my other shrinks?" Resisting these challenges by guiding the patient step by step through processing and reprocessing is vital to establishing a healing environment. For the therapist to assert her authority firmly and fairly demonstrates true caring, in contrast to the empty flattery that celebrities are used to, and allows them to give themselves over to healing—which is why they sought therapy in the first place.

CHILD PRODIGIES

I treated two renowned concert pianists with similar histories. Both had been recognized as prodigies at age four or five, and both had parents or teachers who abused them psychologically and physically. They'd be screamed at for losing their concentration and whacked for making a mistake. Some extremely talented people associate talent with abuse early in life and walk away from their gifts, making it impossible for them ever to be secure in doing what they do best. But these two pianists somehow persevered, though arguably they never achieved the heights they might have attained. With EMDR, both of them were able to heal. One was able to devote enough time to practicing to regain her peak skills. The other was able to overcome her stage fright and gave a comeback performance at Carnegie Hall. But more important, both were able to let go of suffering they had carried for decades.

When a son has extraordinary talent on the baseball diamond or a daughter is a prodigy on the tennis court, parents may unwittingly push the child for their own personal reasons. Recently a top draft choice in the New York Mets organization decided to walk away from the game. He admitted that he had never liked baseball. His true love was football. His father had pushed him, believing his son's skills in baseball were superior and that the sport was potentially more lucrative. Whether he left out of courage or in desperation, the young man's actions stated, "I played baseball for him, not for me. And I can't do that anymore."

ADAPTIVE DISSOCIATION

You are at Shea Stadium in the bottom of the ninth, your team trailing by a run; you are at bat with two out and the bases loaded. The pitcher is famous for his 97-m.p.h. fastball and a streak of wildness. There are fifty thousand people in the stands, and millions more are watching on television or listening on the radio. What you do at this moment will be reported to millions more on tonight's news broadcasts and in tomorrow's newspapers. How can you possibly perform under such pressure?

You have to adaptively dissociate—to shut out not only the

crowds but also any thoughts of failure or success. You have to be able to focus completely on the pitcher and his fastball, to be in that moment that lasts a millisecond. Some athletes speak of being able to "feed off the crowd": they can let the crowd in like water from a spigot, but they're able to shut it off when the key moment arrives.

Professional athletes are truly exceptional people, not only in strength (shake a pro's hand, and you'll feel the power in the shoulder and arm) but in their hand-eye coordination and their mental acuity. Performing at a top level day after day means being able to shake off past mistakes (yesterday's blown play must be forgotten today), the constant scrutiny, the fact that your contract is time-limited, or the fact that your wife is about to leave you for a rival team's pitcher. You *have* to dissociate, or you will fail.

The capacity to creatively and adaptively dissociate is essential to any performance, on any level. The necessity is only magnified when it gets up to professional performing. The concert pianist, the actor, the trial attorney, and the surgeon all must learn to achieve high levels of focus, or they will be unable to maximize their abilities. In this state of absorption, a performer might be oblivious to the screeching tires and sirens of a nearby police chase.

But adaptive dissociation usually doesn't happen without maladaptive dissociation—and some suffer more than others. I once treated a baseball player who was in an intractable slump. We went through the EMDR protocol. "Where do you feel it in your body?" I asked him. "It's in my stomach . . . but I don't feel it," he answered. (Translation: "I'm dissociated from my body.") It turned out that his father had been brutal to him, and the dissociation that developed became his protection. He was fine when he was hitting well, but when things went badly, his slumps were prolonged and painful. Finally, he sought me out. The slump was connected to his perception of himself. "I can't hide it. I really am worthless." In the first EMDR session, he regained his enthusiasm, and in the second, his confidence returned. He went on a hitting streak that lasted six weeks. I don't attribute all of it to EMDR, since he would have broken out of the slump eventually. But the effect of the sessions could be seen immediately.

PETE: BEANBALL

Pitcher Carl Mays once killed a player named Ray Chapman with a fastball that struck Chapman in the head. The trauma of this experience destroyed Mays's career. He became so afraid of hitting someone else that he was no longer effective. A few years ago, a player fouled a ball into the stands; the ball hit a small child, fracturing her skull. At the time, the batter was hitting over .300. After the incident, his average plummeted to .225, and his fielding, until then impeccable, deteriorated into a slew of errors. Nobody picked up on it, but to my eye it was a clear case of PTSD.

In the minor leagues, Pete, a patient of mine, was beaned, an event with profound physical and psychological effects. He compensated for it and made it to the major leagues, but he was an accident waiting to happen. A huge symptom in PTSD is the exaggerated fear that the trauma will recur. In Pete's case, this symptom expressed itself three years later in a home game, when a brush-back pitch sailed just past his head. He quickly fell apart, not only at bat and in the field but in the clubhouse, where he isolated himself from his teammates, his manager, the press, and even his wife. He felt hopeless, and the team sports psychologist was unable to help him.

When Pete came to me, we targeted the triggering event. He began with the beaning in the minor leagues, and from there he jumped to a car accident when he was four. The family car was rear-ended, hit the side of a bridge, and tipped on its side so that all he could see was the water beneath him. Pete had had no conscious recollection of the accident until it resurfaced during our session, but once he remembered it, he was easily able to connect it to the total loss of control he felt after the beaning. Indeed, if we had processed only the beaning (or if we hadn't used EMDR), he might never have fully regained his equilibrium.

Only after Pete had processed through the beanball and the accident could we address the triggering event, the brush-back pitch. In five minutes it dropped to a SUDS level of 0. His work was essentially finished. I followed his progress in the newspapers and on TV. He immediately went on a hitting tear, and his fielding returned to normal. Soon afterward, when my family and I were watching a televised game, he hit an inside pitch for a long home run. When the announcer wondered out loud, "What's gotten into Pete?" I smiled. I knew the answer.

FOLLOW-UP

In performance work, EMDR doesn't succeed in only one session. If in real estate the motto is "Location, location, location," in EMDR performance work it is "Follow-up, follow-up, follow-up." Without follow-up, anything can happen. By reshuffling the deck, performance may temporarily improve or decline. When you've opened up negative issues without full reprocessing, there is danger of regression. If the client *seems* relaxed but not enough work has been done, trouble will follow. With Pete, for example, we had six follow-up sessions and many calls when he was on the road.

Early in my EMDR career, I worked with a high school tennis team. The players performed well in singles but had trouble in doubles. At the invitation of the coach, I worked with the star doubles team in a great session that left the three of us exhilarated. They went out—and lost, even though they felt terrific. At the end of the first session, I didn't know enough to say, "We can't assume what the effect of this first session will be. When you come in the next time, we can begin to assess the effects of the work." In other words, I didn't educate them on the necessity of follow-up.

In follow-up, we first evaluate what's changed for the positive. We then strengthen the positive with more EMDR and bilateral stimulation. We review the remaining negative aspects, then continue to process these problem areas, which are usually diminished and more identifiable now. Throughout, we educate the client on what to expect and—especially with performers who are on the road a great deal—prepare them with out-of-the-office techniques that will help them relax both the mind and the body so that they can let go of the negatives in the moment they come up and increase the positives with musical bilateral stimulation tapes. The tapes are very effective if used fifteen to thirty minutes before a game or performance; it helps keep the system in balance, alert but not hypervigilant, relaxed but not unfocused.

Still, the core work of EMDR must be done face to face: in the office or, if needed, at the client's home or office. As always, trust is the key factor. A person places in the therapist's hands the responsibility for doing something that he or she cannot do alone. With celebrities, this relationship has to be clearly understood as one where exploitation has no place and confidentiality is guaranteed. Stars have every reason to be mistrustful (think of stalkers); many have had more negative than positive human experiences. EMDR work allows them to be themselves.

VLADIMIR: AFTER THE FALL

EMDR helps actors and musicians work with myriad issues that get in their way. I'll discuss creativity—a must for all performers—in the next chapter, but sometimes what looks like a simple physical trauma requires deeper healing before the performance can go on.

Vladimir is a concert violinist who recently fell from a ladder, severely injuring his right wrist. Considering the dexterity

needed to play the violin, this was obviously a severely traumatic injury, one that endangered Vladimir's source of income,
creative expression, and reputation. Healing from such an
injury becomes an emotionally loaded process. In adapting to
injury, people often start to move differently, opening the
potential for other injuries. They may also lose their belief in
the process of recovery ("I'll never get back to the profession I
love!"), and issues of guilt and self-blame may arise ("How
could I have been so stupid?").

Vladimir wasn't recovering as quickly as his doctors pre-
dicted. Was the reason physical or psychological, or an interplay
between the two? If in therapy he had simply concentrated on
the injury and his problems with recovery, he might have
achieved limited success at best. Indeed, some therapists might
have aimed only at getting him back onstage—a kind of "best
possible adaptation" approach—but I believed he could go
much further.

Through EMDR processing, it emerged that Vladimir was
ambidextrous, although inclined to be a lefty. At home and at
school, however, his parents and teachers had forced him to use
his right hand. This coercion not only affected him physically
but also hindered his ability to learn. He grew up with the idea
that "there's something wrong with me" and "I can't think
straight." Ultimately, he asserted himself at school and at home,
but it took him four or five years, and he still lagged behind
other children socially and academically, with a burning desire
to catch up. Could he have attained his greatness *because* of this
desire for compensation? It's impossible to say—once he estab-

lished himself as a violinist, the issue was forgotten. But the injury brought it back full force. His negative cognition that "there's something wrong with me" was obviously related to the physical effects of the accident, but it was also a tip-off to earlier problems.

It took five double EMDR sessions for Vladimir to make the connection between his present circumstance and his early experience. No therapist can effectively inform a patient of this connection; it has to make timely sense to him systemically and organically. Once integrated, though, it brings the patient to a new level of balance.

Vladimir eventually returned to the concert stage. His injury had impaired him in a few technical areas, but gradually he came to feel that his playing was better than ever. His performances, he believed, were enhanced, more creative. He felt he knew himself more fully, and that the instrument, a part of him as surely as his fingers and his heart, was more expressive of what he felt. Two more sessions helped him deepen these perceptions.

By providing access to the body system and its vast potential, EMDR can take performers—can take all of us—beyond what we've achieved, to a higher level of efficiency. It doesn't just cure trauma; it touches on the part of us we call our creative selves.

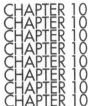

CHAPTER 10 ENHANCING CREATIVITY

Every one of us—from infant to elderly, from file clerk to sculptor—expresses our creativity every day. Whenever we wrap a Christmas present, or dance, or cook, or write a letter, or buy a stock, or make love, we're being creative. The businessman making a deal is creative, as is the scientist, the teacher, the mechanic, the shoemaker. *Thought* is creative. Those who claim they're "uncreative" simply do not understand the full meaning of the word.

When we speak of creativity, however, we generally mean *artistic* creativity, and here it's true that some people—the painter, writer, musician, director, choreographer—are more creative than others. Mike Vance, cofounder of the Creative Thinking Association of America, defines creativity as "the creation of the new and the rearranging of the old in different ways," and Edward de Bono, an authority in the field of creative thinking, says, "At the simplest level, 'creative' means bringing into being something that was not there before." Both definitions apply to art, whether amateur or professional.

I believe that artistic creativity, as opposed to the creativity of everyday life, comes from two sources: the ability to perceive what most others do not and to render it uniquely; and the ability to use familiar things to produce something original. Such creativity emanates from within, generated spontaneously and refined afterward. It requires emotional openness, mental flexibility, and self-awareness. And in all of us, it can be enhanced by EMDR.

PERFORMANCE VS. CREATIVITY

Enhancing performance and enhancing creativity have obvious parallels but also clear differences. Performance enhancement involves shifting from internal experience to specific behavioral tasks. Once you remove the block, you still have to perform a specific task—you've got to *hit* that baseball. On the other hand, creativity enhancement relates more to internal opening and spontaneity. Once you take the block away, creativity naturally opens up and starts to flow.

For example, writer's block can be reduced or dissolved simply by targeting and processing through the experiential and historical causes of the blockage. In effect, the writer doesn't have to specifically *do* anything further other than resume her previous patterns of letting her imagination flow to the page (even though the physical act of writing is itself a "performance"). By contrast, performance EMDR work must lead to specific improvements in behavioral task and function—a focusing and narrowing down.

Another contrast is that those involved in high-level performance are usually externally focused on their actions and may be dissociated from their internal processes, processes that must be accessed or creation on its most profound level is impossible. The concert violinist—or any performer of the creative arts—combines the two (external *and* internal focus) (although how many times have you read that a violinist is "technically superb but lacks heart"; and that Artur Rubinstein hit many wrong notes, but nevertheless was one of the greatest pianists of all time). The nature of the task determines the balance between creativity and performance.

EMDR THERAPISTS AND PATIENTS AS CREATORS

EMDR is both a method and an art form. When a client moves swiftly from thought to thought and memory to memory, that is in itself a creative process. The interaction between therapist and client is an art form, too.

By its nature, creativity takes place in the moment. The therapist tunes in and listens in the moment, then flows with his clients wherever they go. EMDR is so structured, with its prescribed protocol, that it seems less creative than free-flowing psychoanalysis or gestalt therapy. But this is not the case. In fact, structure supports phenomenal creativity. The poet working within a structured form—a sonnet, say—can create wonders of beauty and meaning; the songwriter can take the ABA form and touch the soul. Picasso and Jackson Pollock were masters of line and form.

In therapy, the greater access the therapist has to a person's body system—the body unconscious—the more available he or she is to in-the-moment creation. Healing is itself spontaneous and creative, made up of countless moments that weave ahead in a unique fabric. EMDR works with directed activation of sensory, cognitive, affective, and bodily experience—all in the moment. It works not with what happened *then* but with what the patient is experiencing *now*. The patient's negative cognition is not how she thought about herself at the time, it's what she believes *at this moment*. Activation of imagery, sound, smell, and emotion, and awareness of where they are felt in the body, open the doors to EMDR's creative processing.

There is a correlation between EMDR, jazz, and improvisational acting: within a structure, the therapist(s) riff. A therapist needs a good ear, not only to listen to the patient but also to perceive his tone of voice, its pitch, its volume, and its pacing, as well as the spoken "lyrics" that reveal his core. The better the ear, the more adept the therapist will be at listening to the unconscious and the resonance of the body.

MIND AND THOUGHT

People often confuse the *intellect* with *intellectualizing*. When patients process in EMDR, they sometimes apologetically say to me, "I'm in my head," as if there were something wrong with that, as though they should be feeling instead. But *the thinking brain is a primary part of the overall system,* and thought usually takes center stage in the final steps of healing, just as the body gets the spotlight in the beginning.

Intelligence and thought are integral parts of creativity. The confusion comes when we use intellectualization to deny or avoid, and when rationalization replaces meaningful thought. Intellectualization tends to block creativity. But generally the intellectual process is a necessary component of the creative gift, the left and right brain working together. When people arrive at intense thinking in EMDR, I often say, "You know something? Being in your thinking is right where you should be now. Keep going with it." My clients, particularly those who have had prior therapy, will look at me in surprise. Their previous therapists told them to "stop intellectualizing, stop rationalizing," and here I am saying just the opposite. Thought can serve either as a block or as a facilitator to healing.

CREATIVITY IN CHILDHOOD

Our creativity is most available in childhood, where play is its language. But we gradually lose touch with the creative part of ourselves. As adults, we don't have time for play, or we think it unproductive and immature. We lose our belief in magic and fantasy, so essential to the creative process. EMDR, with its access to the preverbal mind, the unconscious, and the body, reconnects us with our creative selves.

The child who is unusually creative can be perceived as threatening both by other children and by adults. Somewhere between one and five percent of the world's population is artistically gifted. As Alice Miller points out in her landmark book, *The Drama of the Gifted Child,* this gift can be a curse as well as a blessing, for the gifted are often shunned, negatively reinforced in childhood by their peers, parents, and teachers. The message sent is "You are crazy, you are different, you are bad." This shunning is especially traumatic for the gifted, given their exquisite sensitivity.

Some gifted children are nurtured by adults. Others break their isolation by finding a gifted best friend. For some, however, the trauma is too much, and they retreat within themselves. Fortunately, adulthood holds opportunities for suppressed creativity to emerge and for the gifted to connect with others. It's no accident that great movements in the arts (nineteenth-century musical composition, French Impressionism, the Russian novel) emanate from a single group in a single place, nor that actors and writers tend to congregate together. It is with one another that the creatively gifted find a home, where they are free to speak their minds to others who "get it."

Creativity is required for all therapy, but it is especially crucial in the healing of the gifted, particularly those wounded in childhood. Creative people tend to process differently with EMDR, sometimes abstractly with music, light, or color.

I treated a musician and painter who had been abandoned by his mother when he was six. His processing started with the target image of her leaving, the negative cognition "I deserve nothing," and a SUDS level of 10. Throughout the processing, he composed music and painted swirling colors. After four sessions the protocol was completed, leaving no image or distress. He admitted to me this resolution occurred without any words or thoughts passing through his mind during the EMDR sessions.

If an EMDR therapist is not creatively oriented, he may, like an unattuned parent or teacher, retraumatize creative clients by missing their signals and trying to redirect or control them. Creative people tend to process more deeply and quickly; their "leaps" can be dazzling and baffling. Perhaps this is how they were as children, when they were misunderstood and labeled as having "learning difficulties." With EMDR the creative therapist can "fingerpaint" with the patient, unafraid to "make a mess."

EMDR can help with memory and concentration, too. Therapists have told me that when their child patients listen to bilateral CDs while studying for exams, they retain more information and feel more confident. This data has been confirmed by research I conducted jointly with the EMDR Institute on BioLateral CDs.

Adults also find benefits in studying with continual bilateral sound. Hal was an aspiring lawyer who had failed the bar exam three times. While studying for his fourth attempt, he became so anxious, he found himself reading the same pages over and over, retaining no information. It got to the point that he was afraid to pick up a law book. Two sessions of EMDR released his anxiety, and when bilaterally stimulated with sound from headphones, he was able to concentrate. A few months later, he called to tell me he had finally passed.

The next time a name or thought slips your mind, try moving your eyes or squeezing your fists left and right. Bilateral stimulation is remarkably effective in recalling lost information that is hard to retrieve.

MYTHS OF CREATIVITY

The stereotype of the deeply troubled artist supports the misconception that traumatic experiences generate creativity. In actuality, trauma yields symptoms that block the creative process by limiting the artist's unfettered access to the unconscious mind, the intuition of the body, and its sensory receptiveness.

Another myth is that a performer needs a moderate amount of anxiety in order to give her best performance. I think we held this belief because before EMDR we lacked the tools to allow for anxiety-free, peak performance. It parallels the pre-EMDR misconception about trauma: "I'll never get over it" and "I'll see that horrible image for the rest of my life." Yet I've used EMDR to help actors, singers, and dancers to go onstage anxiety-free. When the body is relaxed, connections open up, creativity flows, and performance takes wing.

BLOCKS TO CREATIVITY

WRITER'S BLOCK

Writers who "can't" write hold the negative cognition that "I'm not that good. I shouldn't be a writer. I'll never write again." They become anxious, depressed, and immobilized both physically and mentally. They are blocked.

How can this problem not be trauma-based? Certainly bad reviews or poor sales make it more difficult for a writer to carry on—nobody likes rejection. But creative blocks usually derive from childhood, particularly where the creative aspects of childhood, joy and play, may have been squelched.

Writer's block can be understood from an ego-state point of view. Tess, commissioned to write a novel, felt that she was being blocked by something or someone outside herself. She also had an inner critic who wouldn't stop berating her: "You're a hack writer. You're a fraud!" I guided her to call this critical self into the room, which she did. She spontaneously visualized an angry, scowling fourteen-year-old. Tess realized that at fourteen her parents had divorced. Her mood had changed, and she became frustrated and rebellious at home and in school, feeling misunderstood and depressed. In the session, activated by bilateral sound stimulation, she imagined her competent, caring adult self cautiously approach her critical teenage self. It took time and sensitivity, but her adult self finally won her teenage self over. Tess collapsed in relief. As they hugged, the imaginary teen merged into the adult. The next day Tess was back at the computer, wearing the headphones, creativity flowing.

SYLVIA: THIS REGISTER IS CLOSED

It's hard to imagine mastering an instrument and then one day putting it down, never to play it again. Why would a person want or need to cut the creative flow? We have no definitive answers, but it happens all the time. It happened to Sylvia.

She came to me at age fifty-seven for depression, a feeling that she was too hard on herself, and low self-esteem. Not until four months into our EMDR sessions did she share that she had once been a professional singer. At age twenty-seven, however, she had lost her entire upper register, and it had never returned. I asked her what was going on in her life at that time.

"I was stressed out," she offered, "with relationship and financial problems," but nothing that seemed too profound. Her mother had been critical and verbally abusive throughout her childhood, but that didn't explain Sylvia's loss of voice. For a while, she kept a distance from the subject, but after reflecting on it for a few weeks, she decided to face it.

Although she had lived with this for thirty years, Sylvia had never told a soul: at age twenty-seven she had been raped and became pregnant. Almost immediately she lost her ability to sing. Abortions were illegal then, but she had one anyway, a procedure that was all the more traumatic for being surreptitious. And she went through it alone. Although she remembered the event, her emotional dissociation blocked her from connecting it with the loss of her voice. I guided her slowly and supportively with EMDR.

As she started to process, she saw that what had started as an acute trauma became chronic, and that everything that stemmed from it had changed her. The rape had even echoed with her mother's verbal attacks. The abortion was both a retraumatization and a trauma in itself.

The processing continued. The target was the memory of the rape, and the negative cognition was that "I asked for it." When she talked about it, she felt a tightening in her throat and associated it with her mother grabbing her larynx when she told Sylvia to "shut up." The rapist had choked her so hard, she lost consciousness. During the abortion, she had been given anesthesia through a mask. She had panicked and tried to speak, but the anesthesiologist had held the mask over her face, and she couldn't make a sound. When, thanks to EMDR, the emotional dissociation lifted, the reasons for the loss of her singing voice came together for her. During the processing she made all the connections, and afterward she reprocessed the events on her own. I provided the safety net and the support for her to face the agonizing truth, and then she put it to rest.

After her distress level dropped to 0 for all aspects of the trauma, I wondered out loud, "Where are you in terms of your singing voice?"

She was very hesitant about trying to see if she could sing at all. Her fear that she couldn't elicited feelings of shame, and when we processed that, she agreed to process *imagining* herself singing, hearing herself sing. Once she could do that without anxiety, she started to sing slowly yet spontaneously, with a wonderfully pure tone in her upper register, right in front of my eyes and ears. The moment brought us both to tears.

HENRY: THE SOUNDS OF SILENCE

One year out of acting school, Henry, an actor with enormous potential, felt more and more lost onstage. During performances he simply couldn't connect with the other actors or with his characters. "It's like I can't hear what's going on around me," he said.

When we used EMDR to target the worst of his feelings of being disconnected, Henry told me that he had been a musical prodigy, a violinist who was also proficient with other stringed instruments. One morning when he was six, he woke up stone deaf. He was terrified. Processing brought back dozens of distinct memories, all of them spinning off from this abrupt loss. It took six months for doctors to decide on the proper treatment, during which time he was kept in his same school. Even though he couldn't hear, his teacher treated him like a recalcitrant pupil. Finally, nine months after his trauma, he had surgery and regained his hearing. He returned to his violin, but it was never the same, and as a teen he turned to acting.

The EMDR processing evoked tremendous emotion. Memories of Henry's silent prison evoked sobs, and feelings of terror and disconnection, much as he now felt onstage. He went from deep sadness to rage at the way his deafness had been treated, to grief at the loss of his musicality. Remembering led to reprocessing and healing. And his acting began to open up. His block—the feeling of being lost and disconnected—gradually slipped away. He didn't just recover—EMDR opened up new horizons for him, new avenues of creativity. While Sylvia's creativity was restored, Henry's was reclaimed and enhanced. And their healing lifted me.

EXPANDING CREATIVITY

If it's true that all people are creative, then we all have the potential to expand that creativity by removing the blocks (generally trauma-based) to its expression. I've been amazed by the responses to EMDR from people who don't initially present as especially creative (and by the spiritual responses of people who don't appear to be connected to their spirituality). EMDR opens and connects all aspects of the self, synthesizing the intellectual, the emotional, the physical, the sensory, and the spiritual. Whatever the patient's level of creativity, EMDR will enhance it.

BETH: FOLLOWING HER RAINBOW

Beth, a painter in her mid-thirties, had already been through EMDR therapy for trauma healing. She came to me not to get well but simply to improve as a painter. She had other issues, but she told me that through EMDR she had seen new avenues for where her painting might lead. She wasn't blocked; she wanted to explore wider vistas. Her main strength, she knew, was the use of color, and during processing she started to see new colors, could literally feel and taste them. When she targeted form and shading, she soared, and when she went home after sessions, she found unexpected shifts and openings. Each new session reinforced her gains.

In Beth's case, EMDR took someone who was already at a high level and allowed her to go higher. Just as we all use only a small part of our brainpower, so we use only a trace of our creativity. No matter how gifted or relatively unblocked we are (no one is *totally* unblocked), creativity can be enhanced. EMDR is a wonderful way to enhance it.

In exploring creativity, we may discover an existential meaning and purpose for our artistry, rising to a level beyond our conscious awareness. Artistry entails travel beyond our limitations. Painting is one such journey; music and writing are others. And acting is a unique fourth.

CHAPTER 11
CHAPTER 11
CHAPTER 11
CHAPTER 11
CHAPTER 11
CHAPTER 11
CHAPTER 11
CHAPTER 11 NEW ACTORS WORKSHOP:
EMDR AND THE ACTOR

Actors are the people most responsive to EMDR. Actually, this isn't surprising, since acting training is so experiential, emotional, and body-based. To create a character, actors must open themselves and plunge deep inside themselves to activate emotions held in their own memory systems. Konstantin Stanislavski points out in *An Actor Prepares* that "sense memory" (his term) is the cornerstone of acting—and the "sense memory" method is similar to the EMDR method. Although therapists need to know a patient's history in order to understand the source of current symptoms and behavior, acting teachers and coaches discourage actors from extensively developing a character's history, believing that it leads to intellectualization and not being in the moment.

Usually playwrights don't provide much historical data on their characters, so actors look to their own experiences as their emotional templates. My belief is that a character in a scene is both a person in a situation and a person with a history that shapes their reactions to that situation. And the most formative aspects of a character's history, like the actor's, are the developmental stages of early life and the profound life experiences that leave indelible imprints on the character's destiny.

Those familiar with EMDR know of its value in helping actors with their personal struggles as well as easing performance anxiety and creative blocks. It is ironic that as a nonactor I stumbled on a way to use the power of EMDR for acting coaching—to help actors get deeply into character at warp speed.

A NEW ACTING SYSTEM

The seeds of my discovery were planted early. As a kid, my parents frequently took my sister and me to the movies, and I was fascinated by all aspects of film, especially actors' creation of characters. My fantasies of becoming a fireman were supplanted by my wish to become an actor—and to achieve immortality.

At home, my interest in acting was just another way I was out of step with my family. Also my shyness and lack of self-confidence inhibited me, so I never pursued it. Only much later did I find out that many actors are painfully shy and insecure.

A therapist has to be an actor, too. In some ways, every session is a performance for the benefit and healing of the patient. As a therapist, I've been exposed to thousands of dramatic encounters with people as interesting as characters in any play. And I've come to understand intuitively the motivation for their actions.

One day on a plane ride to Los Angeles, where I was going to receive EMDR facilitator training, I sat next to a well-muscled, tattooed young man named Evan Seinfeld, and we quickly struck up a conversation. I discovered that he was the lead singer of Biohazard, a heavy metal group I knew because my son Jonathan (fourteen at the time) had watched their videos on MTV.

Evan is sensitive and intelligent. We immediately connected, sharing our interests in music, sports, movies, and our common experience of growing up on the streets of Queens and Brooklyn. We even discovered that we had both attended the bar mitzvah of a friend's son twelve years earlier. We exchanged business cards, continued the friendship by phone, and got together in New York when Evan was off the road.

Jonathan was blown away when I told him of my new friend. He asked if he could be in Biohazard's next video, and I relayed the request to the singer. "When it's time, I'll let you know," he told me, "but you'll have to get Jonathan out here on a moment's notice."

True to his word, several months later Evan called from L.A. "We start early tomorrow," he said. "If you can get Jonathan out here tonight, there's a part for him—and you can be in it, too."

I tried to play it cool by letting Jonathan's excitement supplant mine, but my long-forgotten acting blood was coursing through my veins. We caught a plane that afternoon—only to find, when we got to L.A., that conventions had absorbed every hotel room. I called Evan, who said, "Come crash with us. We've got extra room in our hotel suite." After we walked into the room and met the rest of the members of the band, Jonathan turned to me and said, "Dad, you're incredible!" Finally, I was a hero.

A video set is essentially no different from a movie set, and when I first entered this one, I felt a childhood sense of excitement. My role was that of an evil, mad scientist out to control Evan and the band with authoritarian repression. It was a *1984*, Big-Brother-Is-Watching-You situation. I was behind a glass partition turning knobs on a panel, trying to control the prisoners of my experiment. I was unable to break one of them: Evan. My character was then supposed to walk into the cell and identify Evan so two orderlies could seize and remove him.

All right, it wasn't *Hamlet*. But I took it seriously, saying to myself, *How do I want to do this? This is my chance to act, and I don't want to just go through the motions.* To calm myself, I squeezed my palms together, left hand then right hand, and was soon struck by an actor's thought: *What's my motivation?*

The answer came quickly: *I hate Evan.* Then: *Why do I hate him? Because I fear him—that's why I have to control him.* As I was thinking this through, a memory popped into my head. I was a teenager arguing with my father, who was being harsh and aggressive. But my real father was neither harsh nor aggressive. I realized that the memory wasn't "mine" but belonged to the mad scientist. His father was harsh with him and controlling him, and I, the scientist, was replicating his behavior with Evan.

Other created memories started to flow in character: I was humiliated in school, called a nerd by the "cool" kids because I wore glasses and walked duck-footed. So I told myself, *When they start shooting and I enter the cell, I'll walk with my feet sticking out; I'll let my nerdiness intensify the anger and my need for control.*

"Action!" called the director, and I strode onto the set, totally in character. I walked up to Evan and went face to face with him, pointing him out with an intensity I didn't have to feign. The orderlies removed him on cue, and I followed them out.

Evan caught up to me backstage about ten minutes later. "What got into you?" he asked. "When you got into my face, you scared the shit out of me." (This from a man, remember, who grew up on the streets of Brooklyn!)

The shooting continued until three o'clock in the morning, and I had three more scenes, all of which I played turbocharged by my newfound technique. I also had the pleasure of watching Jonathan being filmed—he played a drone dressed in the same garb as the band members, and he followed them wherever they went, both on and off camera.

At that point, I sensed I had created something special, something beyond my expectations. It sat in the back of my mind, waiting for the right time and place to emerge.

THE NEW ACTORS WORKSHOP

Six months later George Morrison, the president of the New Actors Workshop, called me up out of the blue. He had attended a seminar with Francine Shapiro and become interested in the potential of EMDR for training actors. He had a friend who was an EMDR therapist, who had mentioned that I had done work with performing artists struggling with anxiety and creative blocks. Would I be interested in coming to the workshop and meeting with him? Sure, I said, remembering how I had used EMDR to get myself quickly into the character of the mad scientist. We set a time for the following week.

With George at the meeting was Rex Knowles, one of his top acting teachers. After fifteen minutes of getting to know one another, the conversation turned to EMDR. George reflected that a powerful clinical tool such as this might have applications to acting. I suggested that I might have found a way of doing it.

Most people might have responded by asking a slew of questions, but not these actors. It's one of the things I love about actors—their openness and readiness to explore. Rex said, "Let's do it!"

"Choose a character," I replied.

He thought a moment. "Sidney from *Absurd Person Singular.* I played him in the 1970s. He's an uptight accountant."

I've expanded the technique considerably since that day, but at the time I simply came back with "Okay. You're Sidney, and I'm going to do some EMDR work with you as Sidney."

It was no big deal for him. He looked the same to me, but suddenly he wasn't Rex anymore. I was face to face with Sidney.

"What's something that bothers you now?" I asked Sidney.

"Even though I'm a successful accountant, I'm sometimes insecure about my abilities."

"Okay, let's start with that." I had him put on the head-phones and listen to a bilateral CD. "Let your mind go back to an early insecurity experience in your life, not as Rex—he's not here—but as Sidney."

"I'm in the third grade," he said rocking back in his chair. "I'm sitting in class. I've screwed up on a problem, and the teacher is berating me. 'You'll never be any good in math,' the teacher mocks. I'm feeling a mix of rage and humiliation."

"Where do you experience it in your body?"

Sidney reflected, "It's running up from my abdomen through my chest." Then his thoughts jumped to his family—mother, father, and two sisters—and the feeling they transmitted that somehow he would never measure up, never succeed in life. He locked his eyes on mine. "That message has haunted me my whole life."

For the first few seconds of this last revelation, I thought it was Rex talking to me as Rex, but then I realized I was fooled by his acting; it was Sidney talking to me. I asked if Rex was ready to come back, and I saw his face metamorphose. In a few seconds Rex had returned.

"Holy shit," Rex said. "That was amazing."

I thought it was amazing, too. After all, the technique had been purely theoretical for me. Until that moment I had no idea of its potential. George Morrison had been observing the experiment intently, without interrupting us. "You know something," he said when we were finished, "I just saw a guy who doesn't know anything about teaching acting do more in ten minutes than I've seen an acting coach do in hours."

George asked me if I would try this technique out in his advanced scene-work class, and I quickly agreed.

SCENE WORK

I arrived at the classroom the next week and was met by a group of actors performing a cacophony of vocal exercises and practicing lines. I felt out of place. A nonactor bringing them a new approach had been sprung on them with little preparation. They responded with curiosity, confusion, and skepticism. Yet I could feel their interest. Two students had prepared the scene from *Death of a Salesman* when Biff charges his father, Willy Loman, with adultery. George instructed them to go up onstage, and they performed the scene in a workmanlike fashion. George then nodded to me, and I went onstage to do my thing.

"Which of you would like to try this out?" I asked. They looked at each other, and then the guy who played Biff, an actor named Jim, nodded to me. I handed him the headphones with a brief explanation of how the process works. "From here on, I'm talking to you as Biff, not as Jim. Let your mind go back to a memory that somehow relates to this scene."

"I've got it. I was five, and my father, Willy, was going off on a sales trip."

"Can you see that picture?" I asked.

"Yes."

"What negative thought goes with it?"

"I'll never see Daddy again."

"What feeling does that bring to you?"

"Sadness . . . and fear."

"Where do you feel it in your body?"

"My chest."

"Okay, just see where your mind goes from there."

Jim/Biff then flashed through lightning-quick memories of his parents fighting, of his mother crying, of playing with his overly aggressive brother, of feeling lost in school. Amazingly, all these memories were solely Biff's. (Jim didn't even have a brother.) Jim had "invented" them, yet they were a part of Biff's body system. I asked Biff to return to the present, and then I asked Jim to return. He opened his eyes. "That was a trip!"

The two actors then replayed the scene, only Jim was transformed. He wasn't *playing* Biff—he *was* Biff. His eyes flashed, he moved spontaneously, and the actor playing Willy Loman was drawn into his energy. All George could say was "Wow!"

The students couldn't wait to ask Jim what he felt in the replayed scene. "I felt it coming from my body—like the memories were inside of me. I found many moments when I had new choices: how to say a word, hold a prop, how to move."

The second scene presented was from *The Glass Menagerie*, the first meeting between Laura and the Gentleman Caller. In the first-run through, the actors did a great job; to me it was theater quality already. *How am I going to improve on this?* I wondered.

This time I worked with an actress named Ellie. She put on the headphones, I repeated the instructions, and she became Laura. Her first memory was of becoming ill and calling pleurisy "blue roses." Then she jumped to an image from age five of her mother berating her "mendacity, mendacity, mendacity." She flashed through so many memories, she couldn't report them all. Spontaneously she took off the headphones and said, "Let's go."

The actors launched into the scene again, and it crackled, Laura drawing her partner along with her. I felt as if I were in the front row of a Broadway production. At the end of the scene, Ellie sat down, composed herself, then suddenly looked up with a Cheshire cat grin.

How can an actor develop a memory that isn't his own? A trained actor creates in a fashion parallel to a novelist. Undoubtedly the creation is metaphorically autobiographical on an unconscious level, yet EMDR goes so deep into the neurophysiological system that the memories created seem unique, as if they belonged solely to the character.

This first experience led George and me to develop a routine. He brought me into class every other week, students would perform a scene, he would comment, and I would do my coaching, followed by a second run-through of the scene. I soon came up with a new wrinkle—preparing both actors simultaneously, with each wearing headphones coming out of the same CD player, split by a Y jack.

I would talk to each actor in character, first one and then the other, going back and forth every thirty to sixty seconds, guiding them to return to an earlier memory that flowed from the scene.

Focusing on the "sense memory" aspect of the protocol, I'd

ask, "What did you see?" "What did you hear?" "Smell?" "What do you feel in your body?" "Where?" I'd have the first actor process, and then go over to the other and repeat the same thing. After a while, the characters would not fix on one memory or feeling but would go deeper and deeper, shifting from created memory to created memory, just as a patient would do in EMDR therapy. I'd finish by instructing the actors to look into each other's eyes and, without saying anything, process the experience, remove the headphones, and begin the scene again, spontaneously, when they felt ready. As they did, I quietly walked off the stage.

Thereafter I started bringing in more psychological, developmental theory, particularly trauma-based ones. Like people, characters are not two-dimensional but multidimensional. Most of the characters you see in plays, much like people who come for therapy, have significant trauma backgrounds; if they didn't, they wouldn't be three-dimensional. Acting teachers, as I've noted, tend to discourage actors from developing a personal history for their characters, but just as profound or traumatic events define our personalities, the same applies to those of characters. The EMDR-based idea that defining events are held in the system and can be activated, bodily and unconsciously, has been virtually unknown to actors, yet they take to it immediately.

Two students were preparing a scene where a woman flees the wedding altar when her long-lost father, who had sexually abused her in childhood, shows up. She turns up amnesiac, a thousand miles away, taken care of by a stranger. This stranger had left his wife a year earlier, after the death of their infant son. I helped the students understand how their characters' trauma history had brought them together, giving further dimension to EMDR acting processing and helping them deepen the scene.

As I continued to work with George's class, the changes from scene to scene were sometimes startling. The actors might play a scene first as comedy, yet the second run-through turned it dramatic. At other times it reversed, as the humor overtook the drama. Meanwhile I was learning the craft of acting, not only from watching the students but also from listening to George guide them.

One day George invited me to sit in on the master class taught by Mike Nichols, the great director of both plays and movies and one of my heroes. Before Nichols arrived, I worked privately with two actresses in the class on the confrontation scene between Elena and Sonya in the third act of *Uncle Vanya*. (Both were highly anxious about doing a scene for Mike Nichols, and they asked me to do EMDR coaching with them to prepare.) The first time we worked together for two hours, the second time for five hours, and one last time for an hour just before class. By the time the work was finished, they felt that between the two characters there was a long and complex history that culminated in conflict but also mutual need. Both actresses reported a sense of calm; they knew that they were ready.

The scene was a triumph. Nichols knew nothing of their preparation nor my part in it; he was only aware that he was seeing two extremely talented actresses in one of the greatest scenes in Western literature. The forty or so other students in the audience were equally absorbed.

When the scene ended, for a long moment there was only silence. Finally, Nichols said, "That was quite remarkable," and called the actresses over, congratulating them. They told him they had prepared the scene using "David Grand's EMDR acting techniques," and to my immense pleasure he replied that George had told him about it. "David," he said, "would you like to come up onstage with the actors?"

I would and I did. Nichols asked me questions about my methods, and I told him how EMDR can help actors deepen their characterizations. He asked me to demonstrate with two different actors doing a scene from a different play—a minor modern comedy. The pair came onstage. Their first run-through was good; they got easy laughs. Two real, fallible, somewhat ridiculous people were joined in a situation where she wanted to seduce him and he was having none of it. Nothing is funnier than reality (nor, of course, more tragic). After the EMDR acting coaching, however, they were able to convey the humanness of the situation as well as its humor. The scene crackled because the audience could identify with the characters, not laugh at them. Nichols was again impressed.

WORKING WITH PROFESSIONAL ACTORS

Since then, many people in the acting community have become aware of my work, and I've worked not only with actors but also with acting coaches, directors, and writers. Some have come to see me for personal reasons as well as professional ones, others just to improve their performance, though personal issues often arose. For me, it is especially gratifying to work with theater people. More than ever my office becomes a sort of stage, where they—and I—play out our roles.

DAVID: THE NOBLE MOOR

He was an imposing African American actor with a resonant speaking voice the equal of James Earl Jones's. When he projected vocally, the wall behind me seemed to shake. Now he was preparing for a role he had played years earlier, Othello, for a theater company in Virginia.

David Toney had been referred to me by a colleague who was familiar with my acting work. David was seeking greater understanding of the heart, soul, and mind of the Moor.

One of the most stimulating aspects of the EMDR technique is that it is adaptable. When working with David, an idea came to me in a flash to help the transition in and out of character: "Into the Looking Glass."

He put on the headphones and began to reflexively flick his eyes back and forth.

"I want you to imagine that you're looking at yourself in a mirror," I said.

When you ask actors to imagine something, they'll do it almost before you can finish the sentence. "Can you see yourself?" I asked.

"Yes."

I had him process it just for the experience. "Now what I want you to see when you look in the mirror is not yourself but Othello. Can you see him?"

"Easily."

"What does he look like? What is he wearing?"

"He looks like a warrior, and he's dressed in a royal white and crimson robe."

"Good. Now I want you to become Othello looking in the mirror and seeing yourself."

A pause. Then: "Got it."

"From now on, I'm going to be talking to you as Othello. Now, Othello, look in the mirror and see yourself."

Thus we started, with David looking at David, then David looking at Othello, then Othello looking at David and finally Othello looking at Othello. My aim was to give him a means not only for going more quickly into character but for getting out of character when we had finished. With Othello undergoing EMDR, I asked him to let his mind drift back to an earlier experience in his life that was profound or traumatic. Othello quickly flashed back to the murder of his father (a created memory not in Shakespeare). I guided Othello to see the images, hear the sounds, and be aware of his feelings and where they were in his body. He quickly moved to the first time he had killed a man, when he was eleven years old, to protect his mother. These incidents defined how he had become a warrior, a great general, and I asked him to describe what it felt like to kill someone. He told me of putting his sword through a man and feeling him shudder.

That day I had completed a *New York Times* crossword puzzle containing the name Iago, and when I shared this with him, he glowered at me and bellowed, "Do not speak ill of Iago!" We came to Desdemona, and he processed his attraction to her, his passion for her, and eventually his conviction that she had betrayed him. The director in Virginia had instructed David that when he became convinced of Desdemona's infidelity, he wanted him to fall onto the stage and have a seizure (as Laurence Olivier had done in a London production), and he dreaded this moment, afraid to lose control in front of so many people. Everything David and I did led up to it, and when we reached the moment when he would have to undergo it, he said it felt like electricity was pulsing in his brain and that he could smell ozone. Throughout David was wearing the headphones—EMDR married with acting training.

He imagined that lightning had really struck him, and there, in my office, he actually enacted a seizure, bellowing about the soldiers he had killed, seeing their body parts, hurling fury at Desdemona. My next client was in the waiting room, and I wondered what he thought of the screaming, but I knew I could not rush to close down the process. After Othello finished the scene, I guided him out of character, first by having Othello view Othello in the imaginary mirror; then Othello saw David; then they flipped and David saw Othello; and they ended with David looking at David—securely back to himself.

Perhaps some of this could have been accomplished without bilateral stimulation, but the speed of the transformation, the depth of the characterization, and the impact of the memories on Othello would not have been nearly so great. Perhaps David would not have experienced the seizure so that it felt organic to him. Iago, his past, and his own imagination had reduced him to the quivering wreck he became on my office floor—and would become onstage night after night.

I met with David a second time to prepare him for rehearsals, which were to start later that week in Virginia. I guided him with EMDR to reexperience and build on the first meeting; new memories emerged, and again he had his seizure, and this time it was less explosive and he was more integrated with it. He was now an actor inside of a man with uncontrollable passions, not the man himself.

I traveled to Virginia for opening night, and an hour before David was to go on, we met for a half-hour guided bilateral prep session. This might have been a high-wire act for some, but again we were comfortable with each other, and it did not seem risky to either of us. It was David's wish to do it, and I guided him to clear his body so he was able to relax and flow with the session. Then we walked over to the theater together, he went backstage, and I went to my seat.

A great play engenders great performances, and David's was truly memorable. His Othello was a real person, not acting but *being*. I shared the experience with Nina and Jonathan, who had accompanied me to Virginia, and what I saw in my family's faces and the faces in the audience reassured me. We had all experienced something remarkable.

My family and I were invited backstage after the performance. David nearly knocked the wind out of me with a hug, then drew me aside. At our final pre-play session, I had asked him what his goal was. "To meet my expectations," he replied. Now I said, "Well, did you meet your expectations?" His performance was his eloquent answer; his response to me then was a simple "Yes."

Although New York is arguably the theatrical acting center of the world, when it comes to film, Los Angeles is the hub. Recently I went out there to present a three-hour showcase where I demonstrated my work to actors, acting teachers, directors, and producers. The response was uniformly positive; some stated it was "the wave of the future."

No actor can do EMDR on himself, any more than an actor can replicate the experience of working with a good acting coach. But some of the techniques can be adapted for self-use. (I'll have more to say on this in Chapter 14.) For me, EMDR as an acting tool remains an exciting and rewarding venture, and its potential is as yet untapped. It has been a journey to a realm I've enjoyed deeply—one of many journeys, external and internal, that I have taken with EMDR as my guide.

IV
THE DOORS SWING OPEN: MY JOURNEY WITH EMDR

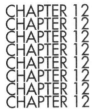

CHAPTER 12
CHAPTER 12
CHAPTER 12
CHAPTER 12
CHAPTER 12
CHAPTER 12
CHAPTER 12
CHAPTER 12   KNOCKED DOWN, DRAGGED OUT:
TRAUMA IN MY FAMILY

A good portion of my practice is currently composed of therapists, mostly EMDR therapists. After guiding so many of their own patients to their own warp-speed miracles, these clinicians say, in effect, "Hey, I want this for myself," and so they turn to other experienced EMDR therapists to address their own struggles. (Psychoanalysts, of course, undergo psychoanalysis as a requirement of their own training.) All of us have experienced trauma at some point in our lives—it is ubiquitous growing up in this world—and therapists are certainly no exception. The concept of the wounded healer traces back to the ancient wisdom and practices of shamanism, wherein the healer's abilities are deepened by being sensitized by his or her own traumas. Facing and overcoming our own deep wounds tends to make us stronger, wiser, and often more spiritually attuned.

Not all traumas occur in childhood. Sometimes traumas

happen to therapists during the course of their adult lives—
major surgery, an automobile accident, the death of a loved
one. And these adult traumas, like childhood traumas, must be
addressed so that they do not interfere in the therapists' work
with their patients. Without the tools of EMDR, this trauma
work can be as long and as arduous as psychoanalysis; but with
EMDR, the alleviation of adult trauma, while not necessarily a
simple matter, is possible in a brief time.

THE DEATH OF MY FATHER

In 1985 things were coming together in my professional and
personal lives. EMDR therapy still lay in my future, but my
more conventional work was going well, and I was building an
active, successful practice that enabled me to make a down pay-
ment on a new house. I was thirty-three, I had been married to
Nina for three years, and Jonathan was one year old. All seemed
right in my world.

But my father was struggling with a number of undiagnosed
physical symptoms. He suffered constant lower back pain,
whose source no medical expert could find. The doctors put
him through a regimen of physical therapy that did nothing to
alleviate his discomfort. He had a bulge in his upper chest that
was diagnosed as a pulled muscle. Finally, they decided to send
him for a CAT scan.

I don't know if this happens to other therapists, but it seems
that whenever I get disturbing news, I'm in the office, in session. I don't answer my phone when I'm with a patient, but

when the session is over, as a rule, I check my messages. My wife has a special code for an emergency: three single rings, each followed by a hang-up. It alerts me to call her ASAP. If she tells me bad news that I can do nothing about immediately, I digest it and try to go on with my work to the best of my ability. On the rare occasions I am faced with a personal emergency, I cancel my appointments and attend to the problem.

On this day I got a call from my parents at their home. My father was on one phone, my mother on the extension. My mother was crying uncontrollably. The CAT scan results were in. They showed a tumor in my father's lower back that was likely malignant. I decided to see my last two patients of the evening and then drive to my parents' house. The endless car ride was filled with questions.

Is it malignant or benign?

If malignant, is it the source tumor?

If it's not the source tumor, what is the source?

No matter what, is it treatable?

If it's treatable, is Dad looking at surgery, radiation, chemotherapy, or some combination of the three?

If it's treatable, what's the chance of recurrence?

If it isn't treatable, how much time does Dad have?

My father was seventy-three, did not smoke, watched his diet, walked a lot, and in general took pretty good care of himself. So it didn't appear that a lifestyle issue had led to the growth. Yet in the following days and weeks, every step of the way, the worst possible news came back. The tumor was malignant. It had spread. It was kidney cancer, which was virtually incurable when metastasized. When my sister Debbie and I spoke to the surgeon, he announced—in that "frank" but cruel way that some doctors consider proper bedside manner—"Don't get your hopes up. My mother-in-law had the same kind of cancer. She was gone in three months."

One of the factors that helps people persevere is hope. But this surgeon's news and his method of delivery—he hadn't told my parents yet—dashed our hope right away. My mother took it hardest when she was told; she almost passed out. As for my father, it wasn't clear how much he was in touch with his feelings because he certainly didn't share them. Dad was philosophical, showing his strength of character throughout the process. He provided a good role model with his courage and perseverance. I hope that when it's my turn, I will be able to summon up the same quiet wisdom and, at times, good humor that he shared with all of us.

My father hung on for two years after the diagnosis, not the three-to-six-month sentence pronounced by the doctors. At the time there was no treatment for metastasized renal cancer, so he went through a battery of three different experimental protocols. Whether his extended survival had anything to do with these treatments, we really don't know. My father wanted to live as long as he could, and being able to stay home under my mother's care certainly helped him.

In his own way, he fared better than any of us, for one by one the other members of my family began to break down. Not surprisingly, my mother faltered first. In one episode, she was so overwhelmed that she became completely dissociative, briefly losing touch with what was going on around her. Thank God her traumatic symptoms were only temporary, yet they were still heartbreaking to observe.

My sister also suffered. She became depressed, anxious, and briefly unable to function. And during this time, I found myself thinking, *How am I holding up? Am I going to break down? When am I going to break down?*

It happened just a month before Dad passed. I was moving a heavy chair in the house, when my back suddenly locked in spasm between my shoulder blades. It was as though my upper back muscles had formed into a clenched, solid fist that would not release. The pain was excruciating; muscle relaxants, electric stimulation, massage—nothing helped. I realized that because I had absolutely no control over my father's impending death or the difficulties my mother and sister were experiencing, my body was expressing my pain and simultaneously holding on for dear life.

Three months later I was still in agony. I followed my doctor's recommendations and went in for a scan—an MRI. The results came back negative. Everything was okay.

The doctor called me with the results. But even though they were encouraging, I immediately felt a jab in my right temple, which quickly became a full-blown migraine—my first one in ten years. In minutes I found myself lying in a dark, silent room waiting for the vomiting that would lead to hours of sleep and relief.

Then at 8:14 in the morning of January 15, 1987, my mother called (for once I was at home) to say my father couldn't move. He had suffered what two hours later was described as a "spinal stroke." I sped to their house, arriving just as Dad was being loaded into the back of an ambulance. I followed close behind as it carried my father to New York Hospital. The doctor asked Mom and me to sign a DNR ("do not resuscitate"), and we complied—no heroic measures were to be taken to prolong Dad's life.

We called my sister, who was out of town, and she rushed to the hospital. There the three of us supported each other. At one point, the orderlies were wheeling Dad on a gurney, with me at his side holding a cup of ice, which my father drank through a bent, flexible straw. I carried this memory for many years. As I saw him being set up in a room, I knew he was never coming home. His valiant fight was over, and he knew it, too. He surrendered gracefully and slipped away. Words can't convey what it felt like to be present at his end while embracing my remaining family members. We recited the Kaddish, the Jewish prayer for the dead, and said a final good-bye.

None of this is unusual—in one form or another, it happens to countless families every day. Nothing bizarre happened; there were no "surprises." Yet each of us experiences loss in his or her own way—it evokes emotions that are simultaneously individual and universal. My family went through its own mourning process, and gradually we recovered. My special concern at the time was Jonathan, age three. I was worried about the effect of Grandpa's deterioration and death on him, and I tried to protect him as best I could. In turn I found him a source of solace; his lively innocence was a refreshing antidote to the unhappiness that surrounded me and that I felt myself.

During this time, I sought therapeutic help. The woman I wanted to consult was on vacation, so instead I saw the therapist covering her practice: a mature, well-trained woman who interpreted my wish to focus on my crisis and to take it session to session as resistance to regular therapy. No matter how much I stressed my needs, she wouldn't back off, and I left before losing my temper. I know that a therapist needs to exert some control of sessions, but this woman wanted to dictate the terms. Not only was she not empathetic, she was downright hostile—at least, that's how I experienced it. (Much later I recognized it as a powerful learning opportunity: precisely how *not* to conduct myself. EMDR puts more control in the patient's hands; the therapy can be taken session to session. In effect, the need can dictate the schedule, not just the therapist. Built into the EMDR process is an openness that is in direct opposition to commonplace therapeutic mentality: Wednesdays at one P.M. in perpetuity.)

I tried two other therapists, both with disappointing results. The first was empathic enough but not particularly insightful. The second was only marginally better. So I decided to get by on my own—an old, familiar pattern from childhood. I was, of course, continuing to see patients in my practice, which provided me with a haven from my chaotic life circumstances. The three-year process from initial diagnosis to the completion of mourning (and some aspect of mourning never truly ends) was a grinding, day-to-day, moment-to-moment trauma that left certain wounds unhealed for me. Although the process of my father's death, especially the events of the day he died, stay with me in many ways, I have worked through most of the associ-

ated traumatic aspects in my own subsequent EMDR treatment.

The overall circumstance promoted my personal growth. I
am more able to face the natural and inevitable losses that
accompany death and dying. During my father's illness, I visited my parents weekly, and we grew closer. We never passed
certain of his barriers, yet I accepted them. As the end neared,
he withdrew, not only from me but also from the rest of the
world. This is the appropriate narcissism of a dying man, his
province and his right. But to me it meant giving up the last
possibility of being able to find with him the intimacy I had
missed in childhood—an almost universal story in itself.

MY SON'S ACCIDENT

It was Friday morning, August 14, 1997, two months after
Jonathan's bar mitzvah. Things were once again going particularly well for me, both at home and in the office. I was in session when my pager rang, not once but five times. I did not
recognize the number and decided the caller could wait. Then
repeated calls were left on my answering machine. Ten minutes
remained in the session—I decided to wait the brief time until
I was through. Then three rings on my phone, and three hang-
ups. It was Nina. An emergency!

I excused myself and called her back immediately: "What's
wrong?"

Her voice was both controlled and shaking. "Jonathan's been
in an accident, but he's going to be okay. Some bones are bro-

ken, he has some burns. The hospital's been trying to reach you. He's in the emergency room at Nassau County Medical Center. They're going to transfer him to the pediatric ICU. Get here as fast as you can."

I contacted my last two patients to cancel—the next was already in the waiting room—and figured I could call the rest from the hospital, a ten-minute drive due north from my office. Ten minutes? It took forever.

Was Nina telling the truth when she said he was going to be all right? Was he in danger? Would there be any permanent damage—any neurological or spinal involvement? Emergency room? Intensive care? *What the hell is going on?*

It is the total lack of knowledge or information that gets to me most, and I don't remember anything about the drive to the hospital except that I silently and instinctively prayed to God for my boy. At the hospital, I parked and searched frantically through a maze of corridors for the pediatric ICU. Somehow, I found my way there. Nina was waiting for me at the door. She wore no makeup, and the haunted look in her eyes belied the calm of her demeanor. At moments of crisis, she finds her inner strength.

"What happened?" I asked.

"He was riding his bicycle and got hit. A car backing up knocked him down; he was dragged forty feet under it. His shoulder is broken. His pelvis is fractured on both sides. His ankle is broken." Her voice lost some of its calm. "And he's suffered burns, significant burns from contact with the muffler of the car, and road burn from being dragged."

I hugged her, and we stood quietly for a few seconds, the two of us brought low together, then I broke away and looked into the room. Jonathan was lying on his back in a tangle of IVs, monitor wires, and bandages. His eyes glazed heavy with sedation, he acknowledged me with a weak smile. I could have lost my son—my only child. Everything inside me sank, and I silently prayed.

His mouth parched, he asked me for some water. I picked up a plastic cup with ice water and a flexible straw. As he began to sip, I instantaneously flashed back to the same scene, only it was with my father on his last day. Only this time, I was the father and the patient was my son. He *would* recover, I realized, despite his physical scars, but who knew what emotional ones would haunt him?

Only later did we learn the complete story. Jonathan had been riding his bike on a quiet suburban street in our neighborhood with a friend named Donny, when an elderly woman exited her driveway and then proceeded to back up the wrong side of the street, undoubtedly not looking behind her. Somehow she missed Donny—he and Jonathan were side by side, within one foot of each other—but she hit Jonathan, knocked him down, and dragged him and his bike forty feet, both wedged underneath her back bumper. She backed into another driveway, covered with gravel, and finally came to a stop, at first oblivious to Donny's screams or to what she had done. Her husband in the passenger seat also had no idea what had happened.

Alerted, the woman jumped out, leaving the motor running.

Jonathan was still trapped underneath on the driveway, the severity of his burns on his side and rear end increasing from contact with the muffler as it grew hotter and hotter. Finally a neighbor rushed out of his house and turned off the ignition. He had brought a jack with him and was able to raise the car, having the good sense not to try to move Jonathan from where he lay. Ironically, if my son had been wearing a helmet—a rule of ours that he had disobeyed—the compression on his head between the car and the road might have crushed his skull or resulted in a broken neck or spine. Jonathan later said he had prayed silently to God while he was under the car, asking Him to let him live; he then felt bathed by a warm protective light.

Donny's father, who lives a few blocks from us, ran over to our house and told Nina, "You've got to come. Jonathan's been hit by a car."

"Is he okay?" she asked.

"I don't know," he answered—which meant that from the moment he showed up until she got to the accident scene, she did not know whether Jonathan was alive or dead, a huge component of her own trauma.

The police arrived quickly and took over. Jonathan was placed in an ambulance and rushed to the hospital.

As for the perpetrator of the accident, the car was not impounded for investigation, and she was never even given a ticket. The couple hid and perhaps destroyed the evidence, for the car disappeared, never to be seen again. It's understandable to want to protect yourself, but it's also appropriate to be a human being. To me the behavior of both husband and wife demonstrated a lack of responsibility and decency so great that for years afterward I had fantasies of renting a truck, driving it onto their lawn, and backing it through their plate glass window into their living room. I had no desire to kill them, just to give them a taste of the terror they had put Jonathan through. The urge ultimately passed, but as I write this, the notion still holds some appeal.

The situation was strikingly similar to crises I'd treated in patients for many months and years. (I was reminded of it forcefully when Al and Tipper Gore spoke from their hearts about their son being hit by a car.) Jonathan was hospitalized for the next three weeks and never left the intensive care unit. A screw was surgically implanted in his ankle, but his burns were the real problem. (Thankfully Nassau County Medical Center has one of the best burn units in the country.) Day after day the graft areas required sterilization and washing, using a technique called conscious sedation. Although Jonathan was not aware of what was happening, Nina and I could hear his screams and moans, which were almost unbearable. Throughout, Jonathan showed a great deal of courage. But I was carrying not only his trauma but also my own and Nina's and the rest of the family's.

Nina and I alternated staying with Jonathan around the clock, Nina during the day and I at night. Jonathan's room had a lean-back chair, and I would sleep on it when Jonathan slept. Here I felt a spiritual peace I had never known before. Simply being there for him, being there *with* him, was extraordinary. I couldn't say I was happy, but for those hours I felt in an altered

state, at one with my child. I couldn't even share it with Nina—
we saw each other mostly on the run—and I wondered whether
she was going through a similar experience. One thing was
sure: we both were doing what we wanted to do for our son.

Jonathan had to deal with countless medical procedures. He
had a phobia about needles (he still does), and here he was with
IVs coming out of his hands and feet and forced to undergo
endless blood tests. He handled it all. As the teenage child of an
EMDR therapist, he had shunned any experience with the
process. He'd hear me talking about it to a colleague on the
phone and announce he wanted nothing to do with it. "Don't
give me that EMDR crap" is the way he elegantly put it. At the
hospital, though, he asked me to "do EMDR" on his feet to
help him relax and cope with the pain. I massaged them left
and right over and over, to the point of exhaustion. Sometimes
he would insist I go on even though I couldn't. And at night we
both wore headphones, which helped us relax and fall asleep.

I'm convinced that bilaterally massaging Jonathan's feet not
only helped him emotionally but also aided his physical healing. And he did heal quickly. Plastic surgery may eventually
cover the scars that are left on his arm and side. So far he has
refused it, although this may change when he gets older. His
recovery is now under his control, and though I'd like him to
have the surgery because I think it would be better for him in
the long run, I hold back my opinion and leave the choice in
his hands.

I assiduously avoided doing any trauma work with him. I'm
his father, not his therapist, and the fact was, I was traumatized

myself. I needed to attend to my own PTSD rather than his, and to have my therapy done by an expert. So the left–right foot massages I gave him, and the bilateral music CDs, were solely to help him be more comfortable facing the daily assault that his body and emotions were under.

The bilateral stimulation made a big difference for him in his ability to cope, in the healing process, in his ease with his own body, and in his spiritual growth. When we finally came home, he had trouble walking because of his ankle, so he hobbled with a walker like an old man. We provided him with a hospital bed, and gradually, over the next six weeks, he grew well enough to move on his own and then, blessedly for us all, to return to school and a normal life.

My old friend Uri treated him with EMDR. He knew Jonathan but had enough distance from him to be an objective therapist, and I trusted him. In three sessions, Jonathan's PTSD, the real trauma, was gone. He still had scars on his arm, his side, and his rear end, but the emotional scars were healed.

At later points, other psychological issues came up. Jonathan had an anniversary reaction a year later to the day; he woke up with anxiety after having nightmares and was hesitant to get into a car. Further work with Uri processed these quickly and, I believe, completely. One of the fascinating by-products of the experience was that during the next year Jonathan, who was always a creative, gifted child, spontaneously began writing poetry. It was not about the accident but about his life, his thoughts, and his feelings. The words poured out of him at his computer. Once in a lecture I presented on creativity, I handed out some of Jonathan's poems and some of my own. One woman raised her hand. "Your poems are good," she said, "but Jonathan's are *great*." I had no problem taking that as a compliment.

Nina had some sessions with Uri as well, but I, too close a friend of his, went instead to a therapist named Carol Forgash. In five sessions with her, my PTSD was relieved. Indeed, my most profound gratitude for EMDR is that it not only healed Jonathan emotionally but enabled us all to heal as a family. These experiences completed a circle for me in the life-changing force of EMDR. It further deepened my EMDR healing skills as well.

Occasionally we talk about the accident, not a lot but sometimes. Although I no longer struggle with PTSD symptoms, the accident still resonates for me; it's part of my system, part of my experience. It doesn't change the way I do anything it's another part of my opening up and recognizing that as I approach fifty, time is finite for me, and I have to be more active if I'm going to achieve my life goals. I usually don't reflect on it consciously, but it's woven into my fabric, just like the experience of my father's illness and passing.

EMDR can heal individuals; it has healed my family. And in the healing of individuals lies the possibility of healing communities and even nations. Don't tell me it's too idealistic. I've seen it happen in Northern Ireland.

CHAPTER 13
CHAPTER 13
CHAPTER 13
CHAPTER 13
CHAPTER 13
CHAPTER 13
CHAPTER 13
CHAPTER 13 TURNING THE WORST OF TIMES

INTO THE BEST OF TIMES

My volunteer work with the EMDR Humanitarian Assistance Programs (HAP) changed my life—and again I have Francine Shapiro to thank.

EMDR came into being thirteen years ago. Within two years, Dr. Shapiro had training programs started across the country. Today some forty thousand therapists have been trained in EMDR, approximately thirty thousand of whom are in the United States, with the rest in Canada, Europe, South America, Australia, the Middle East, South Africa, and Asia.

If the discovery of EMDR was her phase one, the development of the treatment method phase two, and the trainings phase three, then phase four was envisioning the humanitarian application of EMDR—seeing the *imperative* to use it not only for the good of individuals in need but for the healing of communities and even nations. In this phase, as well as the first three, Dr. Shapiro's actions show her as a role model, a mentor, and a force for good both nationally and internationally.

THE ORIGINS OF THE HUMANITARIAN ASSISTANCE PROGRAMS (HAP)

The use of EMDR in response to wide-scale disaster began after Hurricane Andrew had devastated Homestead, Florida, in 1992. When I drove by the town in 1993, it was still flattened. I could barely imagine the scene one year earlier, as well as the terror and the pervasive trauma.

Inspired by Francine Shapiro, a small band of EMDR therapists volunteered to provide EMDR for the devastated local residents, as well as trauma relief for the rescue workers, who were looking nonstop for survivors and helping the injured and the displaced.

HAP was a natural outgrowth of the volunteer support provided by EMDR therapists, who now perform pro bono EMDR trainings for local therapists in places where training would not normally be available. By supporting the local helpers, who are best at aiding their own, this approach avoids the pitfall of paternalism—as the old saying goes, don't send food to people, teach them how to farm. Pilot projects began in South America and the Balkan countries, but HAP truly came into its own in the aftermath of the Oklahoma City bombing in 1995, when scores of volunteer EMDR therapists were brought in to train local therapists and provide crisis counseling to a whole city suffering from PTSD. Other crisis teams went in, but EMDR was the only clinical method that was actively involved, most likely because it works so quickly, at warp speed, particularly on recent trauma, and is so effective on the spot.

HAP is simply an outgrowth of the treatment model. It exists because EMDR works even on trauma as shattering as the Oklahoma City bombing—in cases that previously would have left survivors scarred for life. I know, because I've repeatedly seen proof both here and outside the United States.

THE CYCLE OF VIOLENCE

A boy is abused. In adulthood, he repeats the pattern and becomes an abuser. A bitter dispute springs up between clans. The fighting between them goes on for generations, long after the original issue is forgotten. One group claims territory that another believes is theirs. Battles rage between the two groups until the territory has been rendered worthless. Catholics are pitted against Protestants, Muslims battle Hindus, Serbs and Croats struggle in what seems like perpetual enmity.

The cycle of violence is perpetrated by those who inflict violence on others only to have it revisited on themselves, whether as individuals, groups, or nations. Across the board, all involved have trauma histories. If you look into the history of a sexual predator, you will see invariably that he (or more rarely she) has been profoundly abused. A serial killer will usually have a history of severe physical and sexual violence in his early development. When children shoot other children (or adults), you don't have to look far to find reasons for their violence. Trauma begets trauma, in a seemingly everlasting cycle of abuse and perpetration.

Fortunately, most abused children do not grow into adult

abusers. They most often suffer silently, subtly impacting those around them and society as a whole. Some with abuse histories have remarkable survival skills and resiliency; they are able to rise above their histories and lead productive lives. But out of the pool of those who are traumatized emerge some new perpetrators.

Similarly, a traumatized nation will often inflict pain on surrounding nations. Germany's trauma during World War I and its aftermath paved the way to Hitler's rise. The essence of the Balkan death struggle between Serbia, Bosnia, Croatia, and ultimately Kosovo stems from the trauma and retraumatization of generations dating back centuries.

EMDR therapists tend to believe that our newfound capacity to heal trauma more deeply and quickly gives us a new chance to break the cycle of violence—perhaps to even reverse it. And the place to start, for nations as well as individuals, is with our children, for they are the ones who absorb trauma most deeply and carry it forward into the future. Children hurling rocks, shooting automatic weapons, or serving as soldiers are among the saddest images that we see, for just this reason.

In my private practice, I work primarily with adolescents and adults, many of whom have suffered traumas in childhood. But many therapists who work exclusively with children have incorporated EMDR techniques into their approach, including play therapy. The HAP philosophy is to focus on all those in need domestically and abroad; my sense is that targeting the needs of children should be stated as our first priority.

HAP ABROAD

At first, Francine Shapiro's humanitarian efforts abroad were conducted on her own. For example, she provided both treatment and training in Colombia (in South America), in a rustic center set up by local humanitarians to take in children suffering with cancer who had been rejected by their families. Her results amazed her, especially in easing the emotional and physical suffering of children with phantom limb pain.

One of the first formal HAP efforts abroad was made in the Balkan states. A training team arrived from the United States, and most of the trainee therapists came from Bosnia and Croatia, although two therapists courageously traveled from Serbia, which was in a state of war with both Bosnia and Croatia. Such people not only act as healers but provide role models to their fellow citizens in bridging cultural and religious differences.

The first international EMDR conference that I attended was in 1995 in Santa Monica, California. At the end of Dr. Shapiro's remarks, she talked about the work of HAP. In a flash, I knew in my head and my heart that HAP held a place for me. For decades I had followed national and international catastrophes feeling a mixture of grief and powerlessness. What could I, as an individual, do in the face of such massive trauma? But in a single moment I felt an opportunity open up; I knew I could expand my work to other countries, other cultures. The question was, where to start?

NORTHERN IRELAND

I developed an affinity for Irish music in 1993 on a family trip to the Canadian maritime provinces and Newfoundland, active centers of Gaelic and Celtic culture. In 1995 my family traveled to Ireland, where we spent eight days, and then went on to Norway and Denmark.

One night in Ireland, Nina and I ventured into a pub in Kilkenny to hear a local band play. The place was crowded, and we ended up seated at a table with a couple who, we quickly discovered, were on vacation from Northern Ireland. When I asked about the current state of The Troubles, they offered a few vague answers, but after a couple of Guinnesses they began to open up, and we heard tales of normal daily life interrupted by sporadic bombings, murders, kidnappings.

I didn't know whether they were Catholic or Protestant, and I didn't care, but their anguish was obvious. The worst thing, our new friends told us, was the slow grind of living in uncertainty and fear. The husband called it the daily "drip, drip, drip"; the underlying suspicion of others, military roadblocks and checkpoints, trying to tell the difference between a car backfire and gunfire, the knot in the stomach when picking up a newspaper to read of the latest incident—was a family member or a friend hurt?

As they went on, I wondered if EMDR was available in Northern Ireland. When I came home, I discovered that EMDR training had never been conducted in that country. (I did discover one Belfast therapist who had been trained in the

United States.) At that moment, I decided that it was my job to bring EMDR to Northern Ireland; everything had led up to it, and HAP would give me the chance.

The reasons I decided to direct my efforts there came from more than a casual encounter in an Irish pub. Violence appalled me. Though I had not served in the military or fought in Vietnam (and carried guilt because so many of my contemporaries did, and suffered for it), the news images of that conflict stuck in my mind, in a form of secondary or vicarious traumatization. I remember watching on the news the roll calls of the Americans who had died and wondering why no one seemed to take note of the pain of the South Vietnamese or even our enemies who lost their lives. And almost simultaneously The Troubles erupted once again in Northern Ireland, a conflict whose roots lay three centuries earlier, when the British transplanted Scottish families in Ireland's Ulster counties—Protestants placed in a Catholic land. As decades passed, these new inhabitants developed their own Irish identities; Ireland became divided between the south and the north, and the north became split between Catholics and Protestants. The hatred and strife festered for generations, like a slow descent into hell.

At times I have wondered about my affinity for the Irish people and their culture; my best answer is that it traces from my own Jewish heritage. My people have had to fight for survival for centuries, held together by our beliefs and culture; by placing a high value on family, spirituality, learning, and perseverance; and by celebrating our culture in language, food, music, dance, mysticism, and humor. So, too, have the Irish. In retrospect, I understand why I intently followed the outbreak of The Troubles in the 1970s, especially the agonizing story of the hunger strike and ultimate death of Bobby Sands and his imprisoned IRA compatriots, because themes and images resonated for me like those of the uprising in the Warsaw Ghetto and the mass suicide of the Jews at Masada to avoid capture at the hands of the Romans.

I shared my desire to bring HAP to Ireland with Francine Shapiro. Her response was direct: "Do it." The first step, she told me, was to find a contact on the ground in Northern Ireland. I had no leads, so I made the rounds in the New York Irish community. I went to the Hibernians. I went to the American-Irish Fund. They viewed me as a curiosity, a non-Irish man interested in Irish affairs, and couldn't provide any help.

Finally I found my lead in a woman named Joan Kinnear, a counselor at the employment assistance program of the Long Island Rail Road, with which I had many contacts thanks to my work with their engineers. Joan is a first generation Irish-American, active in supporting camps for underprivileged Irish children. When I called her, she told me she had two psychologist friends in Belfast, and she gave me their names and phone numbers.

I called them up. "Hello," I said in effect, "I'd like to introduce myself. My name is David Grand, I'm a psychotherapist calling from New York, and I'd like to come over and train some of your people in trauma technique for free." If I had tried that back here in the States, I probably would have heard a click followed by a dial tone, but both Joan's friends listened respectfully. Since they were academics, they couldn't help directly, but they put me in touch with a local clinician: Patricia Donnelly, one of the supervising psychologists at the Belfast Hospital for Sick Children.

Patricia seemed interested. If I could bring a training staff over, I asked, could you help me? Yes, she said, but I knew I was going to have to prove myself when I arrived.

That was the opening I was looking for. The next challenge, the biggest challenge, was to raise funds. I estimated we'd need $5,000 to pay for airfare, training manuals, and food and lodging on the ground. I knew that one of my patients, who had been healed with EMDR after years of suffering with PTSD from a severe car accident, used her inheritance to support good causes. I overcame my reluctance to turn to a former patient, and she happily donated $3,000. Barb Korzun, an EMDR facilitator, offered her help and was invaluable in raising the balance needed. She and I sold pins and T-shirts with the HAP insignia at the next EMDR international conference, held in Denver, and Barb turned to her own family and friends for help. Realizing the value of organizational support, I contacted my brother-in-law, Irwin Cohen, who was the president of the Rotary Club in Half Moon Bay, California (one town away from Moss Beach, where Francine Shapiro lived at the time). He got the club interested enough to contribute $500 and, of equal importance, provided me with a list of Rotary Clubs in Belfast.

Bridging the continents with the support of sister Rotary Clubs could only further our efforts. We needed a training venue, and we found it through the West Antrim Rotary Club, a group of distinguished gentlemen who also toured us around their country on the day off between trainings. Northern Ireland is an absolutely beautiful land, and Belfast, despite its negative press, is an enchanting city.

By November 1996 our HAP team of five—three men and two women—was ready. Meanwhile, in Belfast, Patricia Donnelly had enlisted the aid of Desmond Poole, the head psychologist with the Royal Ulster Constabulary who treated countless traumatized police officers. Together they had generated considerable local interest among clinicians, and once word began to spread, the interest expanded exponentially. It even reached Dunblane, Scotland, where ten therapists who had been treating traumatized citizens following a school massacre by a deranged man with automatic weapons heard of our endeavor and joined us.

The number of Catholic and Protestant clinicians was pretty even. We weren't training people who hated each other—clinicians have a universal bond—but at the same time there was an underlying tension. In my preparatory readings, I had learned that you never ask a person whether he or she was Protestant or Catholic; their name usually revealed this information. Ironically, the cultural nuances for the training staff were complicated by the fact that we spoke a common language, yet the cultural differences were as stark as if we were French or Swedish. For example, during the training I was assigned to guide Des Poole in his quest to advance and become a facilitator. The role of facilitator is to watch the trainees carefully during the hands-on practicum and to step in when the trainee makes a mistake. But Des—observing carefully—simply sat back in the face of obvious mistakes. I urged him to jump in more actively—how else could the students learn? He nodded in agreement but went back to his stance of noninterference.

I had to learn that the Irish consider it rude to publicly call attention to another's errors—quite at odds with the direct American style. Des and I faced the problem head-on and were able to discuss it frankly. At the end of the training, while discussing a possible time for a HAP follow-up training, I suggested an early date. He felt it would be too soon and proceeded, in front of the entire training team, to confront me on it. There was a stunned silence. We both gazed at each other momentarily, then together burst out laughing.

We provided two Level I trainings that week. The trainees were very knowledgeable, sensitive, responsive psychotherapists, dedicated to their craft, and appreciative of the work we were doing and of the potential of EMDR as a healing tool.

Our training team did no direct clinical work while in Northern Ireland, but Patricia Donnelly, who had made the whole thing possible, took the first training and by the end of the week had already treated two cases. The first was a teen who a year earlier had seen his best friend fall to his death from the back of a speeding truck. Patricia had been counseling the boy for months with no results, but now, in one extended EMDR session, she was able to help him let go of his trauma and his survivor guilt. The second was a Catholic man who was suspected by the IRA of cooperating with the Protestants, a rumor totally without foundation. He had been kidnapped and told to leave his family and community or face an uncertain future. He came in for his session shaking uncontrollably. With EMDR he was able to regain his equilibrium and devise a plan to appeal for support to a local priest, who had some influence with the IRA and could vouch for his loyalty. Later reports reflected he had succeeded and was still with his family, free of trauma symptoms.

When we arrived in Belfast, there was only one EMDR therapist in the city; when we left, there were close to one hundred. We returned a year later to provide a Level II training for the first group of trainees and a Level I training for a new group, and in the interim we helped with consultation and support through e-mail and fax. Today there are now 250 EMDR therapists in Northern Ireland, an autonomous clinical community, some of them exclusively treating children. A year after a cease-fire had taken hold, there was a marketplace bombing in Omagh by a splinter terrorist group. EMDR therapists were there to aid the injured and the family members of those who were killed.

Now, of course, the terror has eased. Our humanitarian team of EMDR experts would never be foolish enough to overestimate our impact, but we were certainly a small part of the trend toward healing, peace, and reconciliation. We were a thread in the fabric, woven together with many other threads. Our efforts were inspired by Francine Shapiro and by all our early role models in HAP, but also by sister and brother clinicians, Protestant and Catholic, who opened their homeland to us and joined us in the cause of healing.

As for myself, I emerged from the experience with many new friends, and my love of Celtic music and culture now has an added dimension. What came out of this peak experience goes beyond my ability to consciously integrate: *Did I dream that? Did I do that?* I sense that I've been able to contribute to something profound and important, and that the tool, EMDR, is a force for change that goes beyond individual healing. For now, I need no further explanation.

THE INNER CITIES

With so much attention going to our HAP efforts abroad, some of us realized that we were neglecting areas of need back home. Beyond the places like Homestead or Oklahoma City, where natural or man-made disasters easily drew our focus, many areas of the United States have limited mental health services, such as inner-city and rural communities and Native American reservations.

I wrote in Chapter 6 about Elaine Alvarez, who initiated the Inner Cities Project. The overlooked citizens from these mean streets are decent, hardworking, family-oriented men and women living in situations that parallel what we encountered in Northern Ireland. The idea of racial and cultural diversity fascinates me—how people can be both the same and different at the same time. It is odd how those differences create mistrust and animosity on the one hand and add to the texture of the world on the other. Black culture, so threatening and bewildering to many whites, represents to me a dynamic example of this nation's diversity, and I find myself drawn to the idea of doing work in the area of racial reconciliation and healing.

Like so many other communities in underclass America, Bedford-Stuyvesant is bereft of basic mental health and medical services. Yet the bitter irony is that impoverished neighborhoods are where these services are needed the most. Bed-Stuy has a high incidence of discrete trauma stemming from disenfranchised youth and the proliferation of guns on the streets. More and more EMDR is being accepted as a valuable tool and is used increasingly in inner-city trainings. Carol Forgash and I co-coordinated a HAP training of eighty community therapists on Long Island, which has far more poverty and racial strife than most people realize.

In Bed-Stuy, our HAP team provided EMDR training to a group of twenty-five therapists working in and committed to their community. Many issues of trust surfaced, much as they had in Northern Ireland. The appropriate skepticism that people express about EMDR was heightened by racial issues. Although Elaine is African American, which helped to a considerable degree, much attention was given to building trust and dispelling the belief that we wanted to use the trainees' clients as guinea pigs for an experimental treatment. We've had follow-up reports of the phenomenal results of EMDR in dozens of cases in Bed-Stuy.

The effect of the Bed-Stuy experience on me personally was again powerful. The multicultural, multiracial aspects of my home turf play a big part in my thinking and in my work. Bed-Stuy was a natural follow-up to Belfast. Here, too, if EMDR can help in the reconciliation and healing process, one more aspect of Francine Shapiro's vision can come to pass.

ISRAEL AND PALESTINE

In Israel and Palestine, trauma and retraumatization occur on a daily basis—indeed, the rate of PTSD for both populations exceeds 90 percent! Fortunately EMDR has taken hold in Israel, with more than three hundred EMDR therapists. However, when I went over there in November 1999 to give a presentation on EMDR at a trauma conference in Jerusalem, I found that in Palestine there were none.

Diplomacy is always a delicate dance, and this situation was no exception. The Israeli EMDR trainers and facilitators have generously offered to train their Palestinian compatriots, who resist the vulnerability of the younger-sibling position that they find themselves in once again. In the Middle East saving face is paramount, and somehow people outside HAP have to get the training ball rolling for the Palestinians and then, as timing dictates, integrate Israelis with the greatest cultural sensitivity into the process. The ultimate goal is to bring the Palestinian EMDR therapists together with their Israeli colleagues on an equal footing. Suspicions in this part of the world run deep. The healing has to ultimately run deeper.

Still, there is hope. Three courageous Palestinian therapists crossed into Israel to attend the 1999 trauma conference, impressing me with their knowledge and their skills. One man in particular made an impact. His name was Samir, and he worked as a trauma therapist at a mental health center in Hebron. One of his patients was a Palestinian who six years earlier, while working in Israel, had seen his cousin hit and killed by a truck, a tragedy that shattered his life. Despite Samir's best efforts, he was unable to reduce the man's trauma symptoms. I offered to go back with him to Hebron to see if a session of EMDR might help. He agreed readily.

The patient, a proud man in his fifties with a striking resemblance to a Native American, was haunted by the images of both the accident itself and his cousin lying in the morgue covered by a bloody sheet. His main symptom was unrelenting pain behind his eyes, a medical metaphor for the pain of what his eyes had seen. He believed the truck driver ran his cousin down intentionally, and the injustice of the Israeli authorities in releasing the driver following a cursory investigation was unbearable to him. I worked with him for one two-and-a-half-hour session, with Samir providing translation and support. During this time, the images eased, as did his eye pain, and his body relaxed for the first time in years. Healing was far from complete; more time was surely called for, and I regretted not having it to give. But apparently he was no longer stuck, and Samir now had a chance to further the healing process. I gave Samir the clinical textbook on EMDR technique, and in May he attended the first-ever EMDR training in Palestine, under the auspices of HAP, one small step in the larger healing process. To paraphrase Confucius, a trip of five hundred miles starts with but one step. EMDR is a therapy for the present and the future.

CHAPTER 14
CHAPTER 14
CHAPTER 14
CHAPTER 14
CHAPTER 14
CHAPTER 14
CHAPTER 14
CHAPTER 14 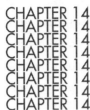 SELF-USE OF BILATERAL
STIMULATION:
YES OR NO?

Is it safe to use EMDR technology on your own, without guidance from an EMDR therapist? The answer is yes, but only in a limited way.

The self-use of bilaterality poses the same question as the self-use of any discipline that requires a protocol and training. You would never appear onstage in a professional theatrical production without years of acting training and experience; even people who act in amateur theater have a director giving them guidance. And you would never treat yourself medically unless the injury were not particularly serious. People treat headaches, indigestion, and minor cuts and burns all the time, for example, without seeing a doctor, but they do not stitch themselves up after a deep cut or put store-bought salve on a third-degree burn.

The self-taught person can only go so far—he can read, but for anything advanced he will need *interpretation* of what he has read. We need teachers not just because they have knowledge we don't possess but because they know how to impart their expertise. Tools can be available to anyone at any level, but unless a person is taught to use those tools—and the more sensitive the task, the more sophisticated the tools—she is best off recruiting an expert. I've tried self-EMDR many times, but when it comes to its therapeutic use, I've found that I'm actually better off putting myself in the hands of a sensitive novice EMDR trainee, someone who has only a fraction of my own knowledge. Indeed, unless I'm addressing a minor issue, I've never been able to work through a full protocol on my own. Something about not having the responsibility for observing yourself is, even for the EMDR expert, ultimately freeing.

EMDR uses the combined tools of bilateral stimulation and the protocol. You can find the protocol in an EMDR book, and you can move your eyes or tap your knees left and right. But just because these tools are available to you doesn't mean you should use them without a trained, competent EMDR therapist. The technique may sound easy, but the practice isn't. When it comes to profound, deep-seated issues such as abuse in childhood, especially physical or sexual, or the affects of war or a horrible accident, self-use of EMDR runs the risk of opening up memories and feelings that you're not prepared to deal with on your own. If either consciously or unconsciously you've carried trauma in your system for years or decades, unlocking this Pandora's box unsupervised may lead to overwhelming anxiety or, worse, lasting symptoms of dissociation (confusion, feelings of detachment or being out of your body, feelings of unreality, or memory loss).

Because of this potential danger, many EMDR therapists, Francine Shapiro very much included, caution that individuals should never use the techniques of EMDR on their own. Indeed, Level I and Level II trainings stress EMDR's power to activate hidden trauma so emphatically that some trainees emerge too afraid to use it except in the simplest situations, and some are so frightened, they never use it at all.

It's true that *caution* must be a byword in EMDR. If a therapist works with patients who are extremely fragile and advises them to move their eyes, use bilateral tapes, or tap their knees when they are by themselves, they can trigger an adverse response. But if they do it in a qualified EMDR therapist's presence, guided to go slowly and gently, they can gradually develop more stability and ego strength as well as more insight into the origins of their problems.

Caution is the best advice in many areas. A person with emphysema or a heart condition shouldn't run sprints, but that doesn't mean no one should run. Caution doesn't mean exclusion. In some instances, self-use of bilaterality can effectively enable you to become more relaxed, more creative, more spiritual, and more productive. The cautionary flag is up, but that does not mean that this wonderful technology should always be restricted to the four walls of a therapist's office.

I use a simple rule: Anything that you haven't been able to resolve on your own for a significant period of time—say, a few months or more—especially if the problem recurs, is something for which you need help from someone with expertise. And especially if you have a history of bipolar disorder or psychosis, if you have a trauma history from childhood, if you suffer from depression that drags on for weeks, from panic attacks or anger outbursts, or are abusing alcohol or drugs, your condition warrants professional help, not self-help.

In these circumstances, self-use of any therapy approach (and particularly EMDR, given its rapid and highly volatile effects) is ill advised, especially if it prevents you from going for appropriate help.

BILATERAL STIMULATION IN EVERYDAY LIFE

When we walk, when we breathe, when we talk, when we listen, when we *live,* we are being stimulated. Bilateral stimulation is a natural, necessary part of this stimulation and as such is relaxing, enhancing, and healing. The walker or runner steps with the left leg followed by the right in a natural rhythm. We hear sounds coming from different directions. (Stereo music is a good example, but so is a conversation among friends.) When we read, we move our eyes back and forth; when we watch television, our eyes shift from image to image. All this is fully natural; indeed, without such stimulation on a regular basis, our neurophysiological functioning would at first suffer and ultimately break down.

Have you ever seen someone deep in thought spontaneously shifting her eyes? Sometimes we're aware of the need for stimulation, sometimes not. A woman wrestles with a problem. She starts for the door. "Where are you going?" "I'm going for a walk to think it through," she answers. She may believe that the reason she's walking is for solitary contemplation, and that's cer-

tainly part of it. But on some bodily level she carries the awareness that the left-right stimulation of the walking itself will help
her make connections and gain perspective.

"I like to read," the businessman says. "It helps me relax."
What he reads may be provocative, inflammatory, and highly
stimulating, but the physical act of reading itself promotes
relaxation, as his eyes dart left to right, left to right.

Stereo music doesn't come at both our ears simultaneously;
one of the reasons we find it enjoyable—relaxing or stimulating,
just like a book—stems from its bilateral quality. Whenever we
swim, dance, do yoga, or ride a bike, we're being bilaterally stimulated. It's a natural part of us, and it exists for a healthy purpose.

The practice of EMDR deliberately activates bilateral stimulation and pairs it with a target that resonates with memory
and meaning. Yes, it unblocks trauma and as such can open the
discomfort one experiences as part of the healing process. And
yes, as noted, this can be dangerous when done with the wrong
person at the wrong time. But if you look at the EMDR
process, the final stage is the installation of positive cognition.
Once the negative has been resolved and cleared through, the
positive more easily replaces it. And the force that drives this
movement, the bilateral stimulation itself, came from nature.

Left to its own devices (unless there is something blocking
it), bilateral stimulation can help us take in things more deeply,
especially positive experiences and belief states. We can combine
it with varied activities, apply it in many different ways. How
and when we consciously use this tool will make it either more
or less effective, but it is always at our fingertips.

As I'm writing this now, for instance, I'm listening though headphones to a bilateral CD—in fact I've been wearing the headphones throughout the writing of the entire book. The stimulation helps me formulate my thoughts with greater focus and creativity; it even aids me in my use of language. When I write my professional papers, I'll often be at my word processor for as long as eight straight hours, listening to bilateral sound all the way through. After a brief time I don't even register it consciously; I only know that it helps me be more organized, more creative, less stressed and less tired. When I forget to put the headphones on, I find the writing more arduous, and I don't like the product as much.

I always use bilateral stimulation to generate ideas. If I've hit a particular clinical, personal, or creative block or simply something where I need to find my way, I just put on the headphones and let my train of thought take me to my own best answer. This often happens at warp speed. Our minds, of course, are always jumping from one thought to the next. This is called free association when used as a tool of discovery in psychoanalysis—and bilateral stimulation puts it into warp speed. With this process come thoughts, emotions, body experiences, and ultimately insights. When you are bilaterally stimulated, if you ask yourself, *Why am I thinking this now?* you will usually come up quickly with an answer that feels right and that can be put to use immediately.

In psychoanalysis, the goal of free association is not necessarily to get to trauma but to explore the patient's almost-conscious thoughts. Similarly, in EMDR, the goal is to get to where the client is going—to a healing point; while this point sometimes cannot be reached without going through the trauma, it can be reached through thoughts, memories, body sensations and feelings that are nontraumatic. Surprisingly, it doesn't matter whether the process makes sense to the EMDR patient—whether he or she understands what's happening in mind or body isn't essentially important. What matters is to follow the rapidly moving path no matter where it goes; the course the patient takes is where he or she *needs* to go. If the path leads to trauma, then that's where it should go. If it leads away from trauma, that is not resistance; it just means the trauma is not yet to be visited. Will the path eventually return and cycle through the trauma? Maybe, maybe not. The answers may lie down different neural pathways, and the therapist needs to be open to following along with the patient, with no assumptions or preconceptions.

Self-use of EMDR technology eliminates one key element: the therapist. There will be no one present to observe, reflect, and guide you as you embark on your own accelerated free association, no one to discuss it with you. Because of this, you must keep the process basic.

EMDR AND RELAXATION

EMDR therapists know that bilateral stimulation without a target or activation usually leads to a relaxation response—of mind and body. So in self-work, if relaxation is your goal, then start with the awareness of where you feel relaxed in your body, a pleasant thought, or an image of a safe, serene place. If something negative or disruptive intrudes, gently see if you can get past it by redirecting yourself to the positive. If this doesn't work, or if something distressing emerges, stop immediately and switch to some diverting activity.

Every night when I go to bed, even if I'm already drifting toward sleep, I'll lightly squeeze my fists, left and right, left and right, stopping naturally as I fall asleep. If I awaken in the middle of the night, the same movements will generally ease me back to sleep. During the day, if tension arises and I don't have access to a Walkman and one of my CDs, I use this self-tactile mode as well. Occasionally I use very slow, gentle eye movements, but I prefer to do something that doesn't affect my vision. The more passive the movement, the less I have to concentrate on it (and fist squeezing takes little concentration), and the more I am open to free-floating thought.

But this is my own regimen; choose yours according to your personal preference. Some people—like the businessman quoted earlier—say that reading helps them relax, but here you may be affected by what you're reading, and the content may influence your response, thus counteracting the relaxing effect of the eye movement.

Many people do choose eye movement as their favorite kind of bilateral stimulation. In self-use, it helps to choose one spot on the wall and then choose a second, horizontally-aligned location on the wall or in the room (a lamp or picture, say). Then, keeping your head steady, slowly track your eyes from one place to the other and then back again, not in jerks but in a smooth, flowing motion. You can perform the same movement with your eyes closed, but some find this more difficult. With practice, either movement should come easily; simply choose the one that suits you best. Make sure the movement is slow. In all forms of bilateral stimulation, the faster you do the stimulation, the more activating it is—which works against your goal of relaxation.

In the self-use of bilaterality, the ideas, techniques, and targeting can be used in only a very limited way. The parent of a child without significant emotional problems can use it to ease the child into sleep at bedtime or to allay undue fears. Children, especially young children, are very responsive to gentle bilateral stimulation. If you squeeze the feet, hands, or shoulders gently, massaging right left, right left, the distressed child will tend to relax. (Performing the same service for your partner may help him or her cope with the stress of the moment.) This approach should not be used if the child objects or in an attempt to deny the child their rightfully held feelings.

If you're angry or worried, the left-right squeezing of your fists may help to take the edge off your feelings and guide you to a sense of greater perspective. A short walk with an awareness of what's on your mind is more effective than you can imagine. At a business meeting, squeezing or tapping your knees (under the table!) can ease your performance anxiety and improve your focus and confidence. And bilateral sound is particularly effective in stressful situations where you can bring a CD or cassette player: just before a job interview, an audition, or a tennis game; during protracted dentistry; or before and even during surgery performed under local anesthesia. During the procedure, as bilateral sound helps the mind and the body relax, the patient can hold less anxiety in the body and cooperate more.

Recently, I had laser vision corrective surgery on my eyes. I had always been highly anxious about anything directly touching my eyes—even if I was the one doing the touching—so the prospect was highly stressful. (As it turns out, I have an unusually high number of nerve endings in my eyes, proving that sometimes a phobia isn't always in the mind.) The ophthalmologist offered me Valium before the procedure, which I refused. I brought a bilateral CD and headphones and played it before, during, and after the surgery. The distinctive whining sound of the laser, the pressure on the eyes, and the burning smell as the laser reshaped my cornea—any of these alone could have triggered a panic reaction in me. But I remained totally calm throughout. (Your eyelids are locked open with clamps throughout the operation to prevent you from blinking.) After it was over, and the clamps were finally removed, the doctor and his assistant marveled that I was the only patient they had ever treated whose eyelids closed naturally, easily. And without Valium!

FEAR OF HEIGHTS

Self-use of bilateral stimulation can help control mild discrete phobias, though not pervasive phobias or panic disorders (where the help of a skilled therapist is absolutely necessary and prudent).

Historically I've struggled with a fear of heights, which became particularly acute one day in the 1980s in Seattle, when Nina and I visited the Space Needle. Approaching it, I struggled with the obviously irrational notion that *this is the day it is going to collapse.* The Needle was erected back in 1962, and it had obviously been waiting twenty years just for my visit to the top *to throw itself down onto the ground.* I wouldn't give in to my fear, so I forced myself to go up, my knees and stomach shaking and my head spinning all the way. Once we came back down, I might have gotten down on my hands and knees and kissed the ground if there hadn't been so many people crowding around.

Fifteen years later, I was visiting Toronto, which is home to the CN Tower, a building far taller than the Space Needle. Having learned the power of EMDR, I decided to try it as a challenge to myself. This time I wore my headphones with the CD playing, and as I waited in line for the elevator, I actually looked up at the giant looming before me. A stab of anxiety came but vanished as fast as it had appeared. The elevator speeding upward was no problem at all. At the top level, I had another momentary pang when I exited the elevator but felt comfortable as I walked around admiring the panoramic view. Then I approached my potential nemesis: an area of Plexiglas about ten by twenty feet, from which you can look straight down, more than a thousand feet down to the ground.

Even though the area is absolutely safe, I could see people go to the edge of it and peer down cautiously, as though they were at the edge of a cliff. This shows what a miraculously complicated organ the brain is, instinctively picking up false danger signals that override the intellect. At any rate, with the sound moving back and forth between my ears, I was fine. I took one step out and looked down without a hint of anxiety. I strode across the invisible floor a few times and then moved on. Only someone with the same phobia could appreciate the significance of my victory.

While I was exploring the tower, a memory popped up. I was six years old and in Paris, where my parents took me and my sister to the top of the Eiffel Tower. The wind was whipping very hard, the railing was low (they've since enclosed the top level), and I was terrified that I would be blown off. The bilateral stimulation delivered on the CN Tower had not only quelled my anxiety but evoked the memory that probably had been the source of my phobia. When I returned to the Eiffel Tower with Jonathan two years ago, we climbed two thirds of the way up (we'd have climbed to the top but the stairs were closed), on steps made of iron grating, where you could see through to the bottom. I felt no fear. One rarely gets to return to the childhood source of a phobia, to complete the process of letting it go. It was a great experience.

STAGE FRIGHT AND AUDITION ANXIETY

For some actors, the source of stage fright traces back to early childhood trauma. Being onstage feels like being scrutinized by an intrusive, hypercritical, perhaps physically abusive parent. That's why emotional and neurophysiological recognition and reprocessing of the trauma are essential to overcoming this at-times-crippling fear. Self-use of bilaterality is not recommended in such severe situations; these actors need to work with a trained therapist.

For other actors, the cause is not so severe. Some may have been humiliated by a teacher or classmates when they tried to give a speech or gave an incorrect answer, for example.

Bilateral stimulation usually produces at least a minimal reduction of anxiety. But it's unrealistic to look to self-work for a complete resolution of stage fright. To expect that is to set up a situation of failure. What I've found in my work with actors is that if they listen to the bilateral sound up to the time of the performance, anxiety may be present, but it will usually hit a ceiling and gradually drop on its own.

My advice to actors and public speakers with stage fright is this. Go to a few sessions with an EMDR therapist to see if the fear has some deep seated cause. If it doesn't, or if a relevant trauma is discovered and processed through, then on your own listen to bilateral sound for at least fifteen minutes just before going onstage. While performing, you can subtly use fist squeezing serially right on the spot. Your fear will probably recede, if not disappear altogether. If you discover that your problems are more complex, then you have to decide whether an investment in longer-term EMDR treatment is worth it to you.

"The more relaxed, the better" is my credo, and accordingly, right before I give a presentation, I listen to bilateral sound while I review my notes. In effect, I'm experiencing both enhanced relaxation and enhanced creativity. New ideas always seem to come to me during this process, and when I step up to speak, I'm focused. Excited, yes; adrenalized, no. I can't wait to get started, because I want to bring out my new ideas. As I speak, I often enter a flow state, where the words seem to emerge on their own; still, I am very present and aware that what I'm saying best represents my ideas in the moment. I'm simultaneously on automatic pilot and in careful control of the flight.

This is, to me, the essence of peak performance.

And even peak performance can be improved. One of the reasons Tiger Woods is such a great champion, for example, is that he is always looking for ways to get better. A golfer friend of mine asked me if I thought EMDR could help him. I felt certain it could and told him so directly. My friend was playing well, but he had some vulnerable spots in his game, especially in rushing his swing when he felt nervous. I had him imagine the situations where that tended to happen, and he realized it happened primarily in the first hole or two, before he settled down. When he processed this with EMDR, he naturally envisioned himself taking a deep breath and slowing down his swing.

With golfers, in fact, I use a two-pronged approach. I have them wear the headphones fifteen to thirty minutes before teeing off. I also encourage them to make use of the time walking to each hole. I tell them to be aware of whatever they're thinking, positive or negative. If it's negative, I have them "walk it off," and if it's positive I have them "walk it in." If the golfer hits a good shot, I guide him to visualize what it looked like, as he walks, and to remember how it felt in his body. But if it's a hook or a slice, I tell him to use the walking to let go of the negative thoughts, feelings, and images. The opportunity for walking in golf provides natural ongoing bilateral stimulation; with other sports, the bilaterality has to be activated more consciously.

SELF-EMDR AND SELF-QUESTIONING

If you're in a deep, lingering, or acute depression, only intensive work with a therapist can help you. But if you're feeling a little out of sorts or something is nagging at you that you can't identify, then self-use of bilaterality may help. Using left-right stimulation, address what you're feeling and where you are feeling it in your body. Continuing the stimulation, ask yourself this direct question: *Why is this bothering me now?*

Your true answers lie only within yourself, and if you're willing to trust and follow where your mind leads you, an answer will come. Don't be surprised if it comes quickly. The more you use this technique, the more you tend to get comfortable with it and become adept at it. In fact, the technique can be used to soothe a number of minor forms of psychological uneasiness: free-floating anxiety, for example, and a general feeling that something is physically wrong even though it's not localized. If you ask yourself *What's really bothering me now?* the answer might pop into your head: *I'm really annoyed at the way my boss treated me this morning.* If your mind goes to the answer quickly, it's probably the truth, no matter how unrelated from your present circumstance the answer might seem. And if you keep going, it may tell you more or perhaps veer off in a different direction, broadening the scope of your personal inquiry. In therapy sessions, when a person asks me a question, I often tell her to ask the same question of herself. What I'm describing here is pretty much the same process, although you are the guide and the guided simultaneously. Always remember the warning: At the first sign of any undue distress, interrupt the process immediately and find another activity to divert your attention.

EMDR AND LEARNING

Parents have told me that their children who use bilateral sound when they're studying tend to focus better and retain more of what they have read. This conclusion isn't based on hard research, just observation of children—as well as their own self-report. We can only speculate as to why this occurs, and it is not guaranteed to work in every case, but in my experience the results are often striking.

I work with a lot of teens and young adults who are facing the SAT, MCAT, and LSAT; with college students studying for finals; and even with prospective lawyers preparing for the bar exam. Bilateral stimulation helps focus the mind while making it freer to digest pertinent information—it appears to clear away the debris. Even with a simple multiple choice question, squeezing the hands left right, left right, will often help you choose between the options. It can help overcome blocks on essay questions, letting you organize your thoughts more clearly. Using headphones before a test will reduce anxiety, just as if you were going onstage. Again, it's all about making connections.

If in my practice I recognize that someone's history works against such an approach—if there's a history of childhood trauma or a clear manifestation of dissociation—then I advise the patient to stay away from self-use before a test (and in fact at any other time). For the rest, however, its effects can be significant.

EMDR AND PAIN

Pain syndromes tend to be exacerbated by stress; ongoing pain is itself a source of stress. Left-right stimulation can often ease pain, particularly when it is stress-related. But proceed with caution: Pain is the body's signal that something is wrong, a signal that should be listened to and fully checked out medically. If the pain comes from the tight grip of a traumatic memory, bilateral stimulation can be a disruptive tool. But for lesser pains, such as muscle tension, minor backaches, and the like, gentle, slow applications of bilateral stimulation may help, especially when associated with positive thoughts or soothing images. Try locating places in your body where you are pain-free and the color that you imagine goes along with it. Activate slow, gentle bilateral stimulation, and watch where your thoughts wander. Return periodically to check on where you are now feeling comfortable in your body, imagine the color that accompanies the positive sensation, and continue with bilateral stimulation.

The same technique can be used with emotional discomfort. Focus first on positive thoughts and feelings, the good things in your life, and in effect surround the hurt area with them— emotionally and physically overlay the uncomfortable with the comfortable. Seeing them side by side can activate a more optimistic perspective.

Self-use of bilateral stimulation helps make connections, eliminate blocks, enhance performance and creativity, and ease minor pain and anxiety. You can use it to feel emotionally and even spiritually more relaxed—people often use bilateral stimulation as an adjunct to prayer or meditation. Left-right stimulation is part of our neurophysiological system that has a direct effect on how we feel in our mind, in our body, and in our soul. It's a fully natural process. It must be applied with thoughtfulness and caution, but in it lie freedom, possibility, and hope.

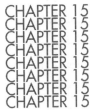

CHAPTER 15
CHAPTER 15
CHAPTER 15
CHAPTER 15
CHAPTER 15
CHAPTER 15
CHAPTER 15
CHAPTER 15 LOOKING AHEAD

So far, EMDR therapists have come a short way—but we have already accomplished wonders. Francine Shapiro's 1987 "seed" of an idea that eventually became EMDR has grown into a tree with forty thousand branches—EMDR therapists— as well as millions of acorns, those who have been helped by this remarkable tool with the awkward name: Eye Movement Desensitization and Reprocessing.

I've used EMDR techniques for eight years, extended them in my own way, seen them heal traumas both fresh and long buried, and watched positive change occur not only in individuals but in communities and nations. Yet I know we are just at the beginning, and that as our mastery of the method improves, we will achieve a speed and depth of healing previously undreamed of. EMDR is the central hub of a clinical wheel whose spokes are the major therapeutic orientations: psycho-analysis, gestalt, client-centered, body-oriented, and cognitive-behavioral therapies. It is all about connections—healing those that are broken, building them when none previously existed. It works to systemically activate and integrate body, mind, thought, emotion, and spirit. And it will grow and change, not in its basic tenets but as our knowledge of the body, brain, and spirit and the interconnections among them increases.

The philosophy underlying EMDR treatment is that emotional change is possible and that individual healing can be effected quickly and profoundly. In EMDR work, therapist and patient together open and walk through a door to the psyche. Neither knows what lies ahead; the room they enter will be new to each of them, filled with the unexpected. And that room itself, once explored, opens countless other doors to countless other rooms, all to be investigated until the patient is systemically integrated and the therapist, also enriched, sees deeper into himself and can use that knowledge in his own life and in his mission to help others.

THE MYSTERIES REMAIN

So already we have gone far, but we must go farther. The brain, despite great advances in our understanding brought about by neurology, both through research and scanning mechanisms, remains mysterious, and until those mysteries are solved, we won't be able to fully understand how EMDR works; nor can we completely demonstrate the mechanisms that produce its remarkable results. As noted, three colleagues and I have been using an MRI scanner to peer into the brains of PTSD sufferers while they are receiving EMDR. We've observed more right-brain activity in the beginning and more bilateral activity by the end of the treatment, but our research is still in kindergarten; we haven't yet learned to "read."

Still, breathtaking breakthroughs are coming in our understanding of the interactions between the body and the brain—the entire human system—that will both prevent and heal bodily and emotional traumas. Indeed, the more we understand how life experiences affect the brain, the more we'll be able to heal its wounds and the symptoms that accompany them. In ten years, we'll be able to cure the effects of trauma more effectively and predictably than we can now; the monitoring of brain functions during therapy (using ever-more-sophisticated scanning devices) will be part of the process.

EMDR will become integrated with other advanced methods that work systemically to heal trauma. Somatic Experience (SE), for example, based on the concept that hunted animals do not develop PTSD because they're able to shake off the effects of danger that has passed, focuses on helping the patient's body, frozen by trauma, attend to sensation and movement in the process of releasing the traumatically held body experience. Although it doesn't foster the direct connections between thought and emotion that are crucial to EMDR, much can be learned from it, especially targeting positive sensations.

Similarly, Thought Field Therapy (TFT) may be able to be combined with EMDR in a new, more versatile therapy. It synthesizes applied kinesiology with the Eastern approach of the flow of energy—*chi* or *prana*—and uses the touching or tapping of acupuncture points in sequence to engender the release of energy through the meridian lines. It's worth exploring.

In psychotherapy as in medicine, archaic wisdom deserves our respect and study. For there are all sorts of approaches to healing the human psyche, just as there are to healing the body. Native Americans, for example, as well as South Americans, Africans, and Asians, work with drums, sound, and chanting, a lot of which involves bilateral stimulation. Researchers, including myself, are even now studying the effects of sound on the healing process. In this new century, old and new age healing techniques will continue to be integrated.

THE FUTURE OF EMDR

I've shown that EMDR procedures can be effective in areas outside of trauma healing. If today it can remove blocks in learning, performance, and creativity, as well as provide enhancement to those at the top of their game, just think what the coming decades will bring! With widespread acceptance of bilateral stimulation's ability to unblock and enhance, athletes may no longer have to endure protracted slumps, and crippling creative blocks may become dim memories for writers, actors, and painters. Students, wearing headphones with bilateral sound for homework or even when taking exams, may find their retention of facts better, and their interpretations of those facts clearer and more organized.

Perhaps even our political systems can change, and the raw profit motive of business, for the benefit of all. Disease, starvation, warfare, abuse, and racial and class hatred—none of these is permanently fixed. Change is now a question of how and when, not whether it is possible. Do I believe that all the problems of the world can and will be solved? Of course not. Nor do I think that we can heal the traumas that afflict our societies solely through the use of EMDR. But EMDR has taught me that things can change to an extent I never thought possible. If it can change an individual, integrating the systems that make us whole, then the extension to our neighborhoods and nations is not too great a leap. Already, in Bed-Stuy and Belfast, we have begun.

A positive emotional experience heals the mind, body, and soul—all aspects of the integrated self. For me, receiving and giving EMDR has fueled the natural progression from healing within myself, to healing of others, to desiring that healing expand throughout the globe. No other mental health approach has directly fostered this process, though individual therapists have banded together to extend the idea of social conscience to larger social charge. But to my knowledge, individual healing has never been so directly integrated into a universal therapeutic approach—until Francine Shapiro recognized the possibilities of EMDR and put it to use in places like Oklahoma City. The healing of trauma, individual or national, means breaking the cycle of violence—and the perpetuation of trauma—by enhancing the cycle of healing. It's a natural flow.

Grass somehow pushes its way through the cracks of concrete sidewalks. Things don't have to remain the way they are. People don't have to live with PTSD symptoms burdening their emotional, physical, or family lives—just look at the hundred engineers of the Long Island Rail Road who have been guided back to wholeness with EMDR healing. And if there are hundreds, and thousands of them, then why not hundreds of thousands, why not millions? We can use EMDR to help heal the world. A grandiose fantasy, but a worthy one.

Over the past few weeks, Bart, a man of fifty, has been coming to me for treatment for trauma resulting from a string of mishaps that occurred over the past five years. He had been in a building collapse; he narrowly escaped when his car burst into flames; he was mistakenly arrested (and quickly released) for holding up a liquor store; and he was rocked in Oklahoma City during the bombing. He responded so well to EMDR that he took to listening to my bilateral CD during his walks around Manhattan. One morning he looked up and saw a man jumping off the roof of a fifteen-story building. While other witnesses screamed in horror, he thought, *How desperate he must be to take his own life.*

The jumper landed on a car twenty feet from Bart and the other onlookers. While Bart was sad and philosophical, others broke down. When he arrived at my office, he was able to report the incident with appropriate sorrow but no sign of trauma. It was, I realized, the first instance I knew of a person processing through a trauma while it was happening. And when he had left, I thought, *Why not others?* Why not use EMDR as prevention as well as cure? It is an area with enormous possibilities.

As for me now, I rarely choke myself from my own emotions

and opportunities—and I notice it when I do. Most of the time I feel clear within myself, aware of my purpose. And I often hear the voice of Bob Marley that flashed through my head during my first EMDR experience singing:

Emancipate yourself from mental slavery.
None but ourselves can free our mind.

RESOURCES

Referrals to EMDR therapists are available from the EMDR Institute (the training branch) and the EMDR International Association (EMDRIA)—(the membership organization). There are more than 40,000 EMDR-trained therapists around the world. They can be found in all fifty states and on every continent. Please note that the level of proficiency with the method varies among EMDR therapists. EMDR training is comprised of two sections: Level I and Level II. If possible, select a clinician who has completed both. Inquire as to when a therapist has completed his or her training and how extensively it is used in his or her practice. It is also advantageous to consult someone who was an experienced, well-trained therapist before he or she learned EMDR. Good EMDR practitioners are like other therapists: They are good listeners, and they are sensitive, respectful, and confident.

EMDR Institute, Inc.

P.O. Box 51010

Pacific Grove, CA 93950-6010

Phone: (831) 372-3900

Fax: (831) 647-9881

Website: www.emdr.com

EMDR International Association (EMDRIA)

P.O. Box 141925

Austin, TX 78714-1925

Phone: (512) 451-5200

Fax: (512) 541-5256

Website: www.emdria.org

For information on, or to make a donation to EMDR-HAP (Humanitarian Assistance Programs), contact them at the following address. EMDR-HAP was established in the United States in 1995 and is a nonprofit organization 501(c)(3) that is funded by private donations.

EMDR-HAP (Humanitarian Assistance Programs)

136 S. Main Street, Suite 1

New Hope, PA 18938

Phone: (215) 862-4310

Fax: (215) 862-4312

Website: www.emdrhap.org

For information on BioLateral Sound Products (CDs and audiocassettes with bilateral sound) go to:

BioLateral website: www.biolateral.com

INDEX

ABOUT THE AUTHOR

David Grand, Ph.D., has a private psychotherapy and performance enhancement practice in Manhattan and Long Island, New York. He has lectured extensively on EMDR both nationally and internationally and has been featured on NBC Extra, on radio, and in the *New York Times,* the *Washington Post,* and *Newsday.* He is a facilitator and specialty presenter of the EMDR Institute. He holds a doctorate in Clinical Social Work (Human Development) from the International University and has a Certificate in Psychoanalytic Psychotherapy from the Society for Psychoanalytic Study and Research on Long Island.

Dr. Grand has taught scene work at the New Actors Workshop in New York and privately coaches actors in stage, film, and TV work. He has presented showcases of *EMDR Acting Coaching* in Los Angeles, Miami, and New York and has also aided professional and elite athletes with EMDR performance-enhancement techniques.

Dr. Grand is the developer and producer of the groundbreaking technology of Bio*Lateral* Sound Recordings used by thousands of EMDR therapists to facilitate healing through the use of soothing bilateral sound. He has also been part of an MRI research team studying EMDR's effects on brain function.

Dr. Grand is the former chairman of the EMDR-Humanitarian Assistance Program (HAP). In that role, he coordinated pro bono training for therapists in Northern Ireland, and he also coordinated the HAP Inner Cities Training in Long Island and Brooklyn, New York.